MAGIC IS IN THE AIR!

Those of us who treasure exotically-scented herbs, precious oils and wildflowers *know* that aromas affect us. The scent of a rose may spark thoughts of love. Bitter frankincense recalls sand-buried civilizations and ancient spirituality. A pine forest, glistening and crisp in the morning air, emanates health.

For the past 40 years, researchers have been discovering the undeniable effects of aromas. They stimulate memories, calm our nerves and heal our bodies. This has lead to the widespread practice of holistic aromatherapy.

However, ritualists have utilized fragrant plants for thousands of years. They've long known which scents awaken psychic awareness, stimulate love, rouse sexual desires and deepen spirituality. By simply visualizing and inhaling specific fragrances, they've been able to protect their homes and loved ones; draw money into their lives; purify their inner selves and enhance their appearances.

Today, the age-old lore has been brought up to date in this practical guide to scent magic. *Magical Aromatherapy* is a unique investigation into the energies that await within common flowers, spices, herbs and essential oils. This is natural magic of the highest order, for its only tools are ourselves and the fragrances.

Energies await within the aromatic gifts of the Earth. All we need do is invite them in with love and responsibility. In doing so, we can change our lives— through the ancient art of *Magical Aromatherapy*.

About the Author

Since childhood, Scott Cunningham had been fascinated with plants and herbs. He long delighted in not only smelling flowers and leaves, but also in releasing their scents and, thus, their energies. His work with true essential oils, coupled with his background in magic and ritual ethnobotany, prompted the research and experimentation that culminated in the creation of this book.

Free Catalog from Llewellyn

For more than 90 years Llewellyn has brought its readers knowledge in the fields of metaphysics and human potential. Learn about the newest books in spiritual guidance, natural healing, astrology, occult philosophy and more. Enjoy book reviews, new age articles, a calendar of events, plus current advertised products and services. To get your free copy of *Llewellyn's New Worlds of Mind and Spirit*, send your name and address to:

Llewellyn's New Worlds of Mind and Spirit
P.O. Box 64383-129
St. Paul, MN 55164-0383
U.S.A.

ABOUT LLEWELLYN'S NEW AGE SERIES

The "New Age"—it's a phrase we use, but what does it mean? Does it mean that we are entering the Aquarian Age? Does it mean that a new Messiah is coming to correct all that is wrong and make Earth into a Garden? Probably not—but the idea of a *major change* is there, combined with awareness that Earth *can* be a Garden; that war, crime, poverty, disease, etc., are not necessary "evils."

Optimists, dreamers, scientists . . . nearly all of us believe in a "better tomorrow," and that somehow we can do things now that will make for a better future life for ourselves and for coming generations.

In one sense, we all know there's nothing new under the Heavens, and in another sense that every day makes a new world. The difference is in our consciousness. And this is what the New Age is all about: it's a major change in consciousness found within each of us as we learn to bring forth and manifest powers that Humanity has always potentially had.

Evolution moves in "leaps." Individuals struggle to develop talents and powers, and their efforts build a "power bank" in the Collective Unconsciousness, the soul of Humanity that suddenly makes these same talents and powers easier access for the majority.

You still have to learn the 'rules' for developing and applying these powers, but it is more like a "re-learning" than a *new* learning, because with the New Age it is as if the basis for these had become genetic.

Other Books by Scott Cunningham

Magical Herbalism
Earth Power
Cunningham's Encyclopedia of Magical Herbs
The Complete Book of Incense, Oils and Brews
The Magical Household (with David Harrington)
Cunningham's Encyclopedia of Crystal, Gem and Metal Magic
The Truth About Witchcraft Today
Wicca: A Guide for the Solitary Practitioner
The Magic in Food
Earth, Air, Fire and Water

Forthcoming

Living Wicca
Spellcrafts (with David Harrington)
Traditional Hawaiian Religion and Magic

Llewellyn's New Age Series

Magical Aromatherapy

The Power of Scent

by

Scott Cunningham

1993
Llewellyn Publications
St. Paul, Minnesota 55164-0383, U.S.A.

FIRST EDITION
Fourth Printing, 1993

Cover art by Robin Wood

Library of Congress Cataloging-in-Publication Data
Cunningham, Scott, 1956-1993
    Magical aromatherapy: the power of scent /
by Scott Cunningham.
        p.   cm. — (Llewellyn's new age series)
    Includes bibliographical references.
    ISBN 0-87542-129-6
    1. Magic. 2. Perfumes—Miscellanea. 3. Essences
and essential oils—Miscellanea. I. Title. II. Series.
BF1442.P47C86   1989
133.4'3—dc20   89-38755
                                                                CIP

Llewellyn Publications
A Division of Llewellyn Worldwide, Ltd.
P.O. 64383, St. Paul, MN 55164-0383

*This book is dedicated to everyone
who ever bent toward the Earth,
lifted up a flower,
and discovered the magic of scent*

ACKNOWLEDGEMENTS

To my mother for all those roses, freesias, narcissi and other scented plants with which she graced my childhood home.

To my father for inculcating a respect for plants in my youth.

To Judy of Eye of the Cat and Linda of Earth Emporium for sharing exotic essential oils and plants.

To Maureen Buehrle of the International Herb Growers and Marketers Association for inviting me to speak at their 1988-1989 convention—thereby bringing me face to face with so many aromatherapy practitioners.

To Marlene for informing me of newly published works in this field.

To Robert Tisserand for offering valuable comments on the manuscript of this book.

To the many aromatherapists I have met—including Mr. Tisserand, John Steele, Marcel Lavabre, and Victoria Edwards—for their research, experimentation and writings.

To Colleen K. Dodt for her generous support and enthusiasm.

To Marilee for her talks in aromatherapy way back when and, more recently, for sharing her essential oils.

To Carl Weschcke and everyone at Llewellyn Publications for giving me the opportunity to write this book.

And finally to the Earth, our Mother, for allowing us to work with her fragrant treasures.

CONTENTS

PREFACE

There are worlds which we cannot explore with our eyes. These realms, though physical, lie beyond all our senses but one. Our awareness of them blossoms only when we call upon our oldest method of discovering the world around us—our sense of smell.

For how many millenia have humans interacted with aromatic plants? How many flowers have been sniffed, roots crushed, seeds rubbed between fingers, leaves held up to noses? Some of the earliest known European burial sites contain the remains of flowers and aromatic leaves, indicating that human beings have long appreciated the hidden world of scent.

We're returning to the powers of fragrance. The resurgence of interest in herbs, which began in the United States in the 1930s, continues unabated. The practice of aromatherapy (the use of true essential oils for healing purposes) enjoys widespread popularity.

Once I'd completed the greatly enlarged edition of *The Magic of Incense, Oils and Brews*,* Llewellyn Publications asked me to write a book about scent. This seemed an ideal opportunity to merge current knowledge of the physiological and psychological effects of

---

* Now retitled *The Complete Book of Incense, Oils & Brews*.

natural fragrances with the ancient art of magical perfumery. This book, then, is a guide to using the energies locked within aromatic plants and true essential oils.*

In writing this book I've drawn on extensive experimentation and observation, research into 4,000 years of written records and the wisdom of friends and respected aromatherapy practitioners. Additionally, I've also allowed the fragrances and essential oils to speak for themselves, to reveal the ways in which they can help us.

This isn't a look at cosmetic perfumery or conventional aromatherapy techniques, but a guide to utilizing essential oils and aromatic plants to create changes in our lives. By correctly selecting the fragrance and inhaling it with visualization, true magic occurs.

Magical aromatherapy merges the energies contained within essential oils and plants with our own. When charged through simple visualization techniques they can produce love, psychic awareness, peace, sleep, health, money, purification, protection, enhanced sexual relations and a number of other changes.

Scent magic has a rich, colorful history. Today, in the shadow of the next century, there is much we can learn from the simple plants that grace our planet. Most have been used for countless centuries. The energies still vibrate within their aromas.

It's my fondest hope that, after reading this book, you'll never again look at a rose, a lemon or a vase of carnations without remembering that some energy exists within their scents, and that to utilize it you

---

* See the glossary for unfamiliar terms.

need only sniff and savor the power.

Magical aromatherapy is an exotic world of costly rose otto, sacred saffron, delicious orange peel and other wonders of the Earth. Once, such things were worshipped. Today, we can work with them to create perfumed futures.

The magic is there. Bring it into your life!

—Scott Cunningham
San Diego, California
March 25, 1989

FOREWORD

In *Magical Aromatherapy*, Scott Cunningham has skill-fully blended traditional occult practices with modern aromatherapy and personal growth. He succeeds because you are the prime mover in this mystical, aromatic scenario, not the fragrances. They are essential helpers, but their various esoteric properties are only given impetus by your creative powers of thought.

In "conventional" holistic aromatherapy, the senses of touch (massage) and smell are evoked, while in magical aromatherapy the senses of smell and sight (visualization) are used. Scott Cunningham offers us a way to create change in our lives by engaging Earth (plant) energies, and making the most of their subtle powers through our own powers of thought.

The book maintains a broad scope of interest by giving you a choice of either essential oils or fresh herbs to smell. At the same time it reflects the need for safety when handling some of these fragrant plants and essential oils. The result, an exciting, new angle on an ancient theme, introduces the universe of plant fragrances in a way which you can easily practice at home.

—Robert Tisserand
The Art of Aromatherapy

PART I

SCENT

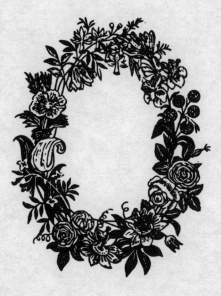

CHAPTER ONE

MAGICAL AROMATHERAPY

As I sit here writing this, small jars of essential oils surround me. I open a bottle—jasmine uplifts me. Another phial—rich yarrow soothes me. From a third, the fragrance of thousands of roses deepens my sense of peace and calms the tensions I had concerning this chapter, which I had purposefully avoided writing until I was nearly finished with the book.

I chose these three at random. Though they happen to be among the most expensive essential oils, I could have inhaled the aromas rising from jasmine blossoms, fresh roses and yarrow flowers and obtained the same benefits without the great expense.

Similarly, when I wish to meditate, become involved in a relationship, increase my financial base or protect myself, I call upon the energies contained within essential oils and aromatic plants to manifest these changes through a process known as magic.

Throughout recorded history, humans have been aware of the marked effects of scented plants on their minds, bodies and emotions. Humans have always smelled flowers, and early humans became aware of the changes specific scents created within themselves at an early time.

When civilization began, humans compiled aromatic knowledge into a body of lore which can be termed *magical aromatherapy*. Certain fragrant plants were worn or sniffed to heal the body. Flowers were utilized to attract love and to secure food and protection.

The rarest, costliest and most aromatic plants were offered in sacrifice to goddesses and gods. Though the aim was to please the deities, incense smoke also affected the worshippers as well. The smoke released from burning frankincense, for instance, directly heightened the participants' spiritual involvement in the rite.

Additionally, specific scents were utilized in magical ritual to attain the correct state of consciousness necessary to the practice of magic. Some odors also increased the human body's physical (bioelectrical) energy which could be funneled into ritual tasks. Other scents were discovered to be closely aligned with specific magical goals such as love, healing, psychic awareness, purification and sex, and were inhaled in conjunction with basic rituals designed to utilize these energies. Such practices continue today and are the origins of the scented oils and incense used in folk and ceremonial magic.

Conventional aromatherapy, which utilizes essential oils and massage to heal the body and psyche, is increasing in popularity as many experience its effectiveness. Hospitals in France are regularly utilizing aromatherapy to speed healing and reduce the pain of patients.

Organizations such as The International Federation of Aromatherapists (headquartered in London) and The American Aromatherapy Association (Fair Oaks, California) have been established to promote this ancient practice. Specialized periodicals are now being published as well as many books.

Conventional (or, as Robert Tisserand terms it, "holistic") aromatherapy is a growing alternative for those dissatisfied with the form of "treat the symptom, blast the disease" medicine. Clinical studies prove its effectiveness in treating many conditions, particularly those which don't respond to orthodox medication.

Holistic aromatherapy is a complex art in which essential oils are massaged into the body or inhaled in order to produce the desired physiological, mental or emotional effect. The art of aromatherapy lies in proficiency in massage, wide knowledge of the properties of essential oils and in their use in treating specific conditions. Conventional aromatherapy can't be mastered from reading a few books and buying a dozen or so oils.

However, *magical* aromatherapy is an offshoot from the holistic branch. It is best practiced alone (no massage therapist is needed). It isn't necessarily directed toward healing (though it can be), and its aims are much broader.

I've used the word magic here to clearly differentiate this practice from holistic aromatherapy. Magic is many things to many people. To me, *magic is the movement of subtle, natural energies to manifest needed change*.

Magical aromatherapy is a specialized form of this ancient art. In brief, the practitioner visualizes a specific, needed change such as a loving relationship or business success. This visualization is maintained while inhaling the fragrance of aromatic plant materials or essential oils. Bioelectrical energy (the non-physical energy resident within our bodies, produced by muscular contraction) is coupled with that of the fragrance and is programmed or fine-tuned by the visualization.

To create an internal change, this aroma-charged energy is allowed to permeate the body and/or the two minds (conscious and psychic—see Glossary).

For example, a person wishing to sharpen psychic awareness might inhale the fragrance of ground mace or yarrow essential oil while imagining (imaging) a huge door opening the pathway to the psychic mind.

Either of these scents, coupled with visualization, will awaken the practitioner to the psychic impulses that they're always receiving but which are usually blocked by the conscious mind. The fragrance instructs the body's bioelectrical energy to lower its reserves, to calm the central nervous system and reduce muscular tension in order to facilitate psychic awareness.

One more step is necessary for aromatic rituals designed to affect the practitioner's environment. Once the scent has been inhaled and the body's energy is programmed, the combined energies of the scent and bioelectrical energy are sent into the atmosphere to manifest the change. It is moved through visualization. (See Chapter Five: Methods and Techniques.)

This greatly varies according to the needed result. To protect a home, the energy might be visualized as rushing out from the body, penetrating the walls and forming protective barriers over doors and windows. To increase prosperity it could be instructed to fly into the air and create situations which manifest additional money. To bring a loving relationship the energy is both retained within the body and slowly released from it in order to attract interested persons.

These descriptions may sound complex, but magical aromatherapy is simple to perform. What could be easier than smelling a flower or opening up a bottle of essential oil? True, it does rely on our ability to visualize, but this is a simple art which most of us practice every day.

The real force behind magical aromatherapy is found within scented plants and essential oils. Once the basic technique has been mastered, this is one of the easiest branches of the magical arts to success-fully practice.

For some of the specific uses mentioned in Part II of this book, visualization isn't even necessary. Inhal-ing the scent of rosemary will arouse our conscious minds. Ylang-ylang essential oil or the fragrance of fresh sweet pea flowers produces feelings of happi-ness and joy—with or without visualization. Sniffing fresh carnation flowers or lime essential oil energizes the body.

Why? Many scents have direct physiological effects. Some aspects of magical aromatherapy overlap its conventional kin, wherein little visualization is used. However, to maximize the effectiveness of any change you wish to create through the use of scented plant materials, *welcome* into yourself the energies which ride on the scent. *Visualize* them effecting the change. *Accept* them as positive tools, and *respect* them as concentrated Earth energies.

Though certain aspects of conventional aromatherapy come into play here, practitioners of that art may disagree with some of my conclusions regarding the effects of scent on human beings. However, this book is based on thousands of years of recorded information and nearly 20 years of personal research and experimentation into these potent fragrances. In its own arena of influence, magical aromatherapy is just as effective as its conventional cousin.

This is a time-honored practice which has only recently been rediscovered, a gift from past ages which we can use to improve our lives.

We can work with the precious scents of flowers, leaves, seeds and woods to expand our ability to sense love within ourselves and to return it to others. Specific fragrances draw prosperity to our lives. Aromas are useful in heightening spirituality, sharpening psychic awareness and creating restful sleep. Certain scents increase physical energy and mental alertness, reduce the effects of stress and guard our bodies.

All these wonders—and many more—can be accomplished through the art of *magical aromatherapy*.

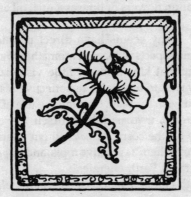

CHAPTER TWO

DIVINE FRAGRANCES

Humans have inextricably entwined plants into their lives. Scented plants have been especially honored since the earliest times. They were used in religious and magical ritual as well as in healing arts. All three of these practices were once central to human existence (and, to many, still are).

The great, vanished civilizations of the Middle East and the Mediterranean glorified scent, making it a part of their lives. Though lesser known, aroma magic use among native American Indians and the old Hawaiians was also extremely common.

The following glimpse into the powers that earlier peoples found within fragrant plants hints at the long history of magical aromatherapy and provides a fitting introduction to its practice.

THE EGYPTIANS

On the walls of ancient tombs and temples lost in the desert, one symbol frequently occurs—a half-round, handled object with lines representing smoke rising from it. This validates the use of incense in

Egypt from the earliest times.

Save for the Druids, more nonsense has been written about the Egyptians than any other vanished people. This began in the late 1800s and peaked around 1922, when Howard Carter unveiled the tomb of Tutankhamen to the world. This sad phenomenon continues, with "curse-of-the-pharaoh" stories and equally nonsensical follies passed off as fact by unscrupulous authors.

Today, researchers have translated many Egyptian papyri. Temple and tomb inscriptions have given up their secrets. Our picture of daily life in ancient Egypt, at least among the upper classes, grows sharper.

They were an extraordinary people. The Egyptians used a narrow strip of fertile land along the Nile to build a civilization unparalleled in its architecture, art and crafts. As Egypt grew strong, its rulers imported frankincense, sandalwood, myrrh and cinnamon from far-distant lands. These fragrant treasures were demanded as tribute from conquered peoples and were even traded for gold.

Perfume for gold. This statement points to the high regard the Egyptians had for scents. They were used in medicine, food preservation, cooking, religion and magic.

Pharaohs boasted of offering huge amounts of aromatic woods and plant perfumes to the goddesses and gods, burning thousands of boxes of the expensive materials. Many had such impressive feats recorded in stone. Rameses III, perhaps the most lavish of the pharaohs, offered 246 measures and 82 bundles of cinnamon on one occasion, and on yet another 3,036 logs of the same rare spice. Such acts of religious faith taxed the royal treasury.

Hatshepsut (*circa* 1500 B.C.E.), described as the "most energetic" of Egypt's queens, launched her famous expedition to the land of Punt, seeking out myrrh and other spices used to honor the deities. Like earlier Egyptian rulers, she didn't come back empty-handed.

Use of fragrance even extended after death. Embalmed bodies were anointed with scented unguents, and jars of perfume were sealed in the tombs for use during the deceased's after-life.

Aromatic plant materials were given as state tribute, were donated to specific temples and were kept on altars in alabaster, diorite and turquoise containers as offerings to the gods and goddesses.

Each morning, statues of the deities were anointed by the priests with scented oils. Incense was burned in many temple activities, during the crowning of pharaohs and for religious rituals. It was also smouldered at funerals to waft negative spirits from the mummified body.

Pliny, in his *Natural History*, recorded the recipe for an Egyptian perfume used during Graeco-Roman times. *Metopium* consisted of cardamom, rush, reed, honey, wine, myrrh, galbanum and terebinth, among other ingredients.

Because the Egyptians hadn't discovered the art of distillation, by which all true perfumes are made, they created such a perfume by soaking plant materials in oils or fats. Olive oil and the oil of balanos (*Balanites aegyptica*) seem to have been preferred. The oil slowly absorbed the scent, creating the perfume. This was the only type of liquid fragrance used in early times—no true essential oils were available.

Undoubtedly the most famous Egyptian incense was *kyphi*. Dioscorides, Plutarch, Galen and Loret all mentioned it in their writings. The recipes differ as to the specific ingredients included. This may be due to regional differences, supply problems, faulty translations or other reasons.

However, we know that kyphi contained at least some of the following ingredients (Plutarch lists 16):

Honey	Saffron
Wine	Cardamom
Raisins	Cyperus
Calamus	Sweet Acacia
Cinnamon	Rhodium
Juniper	Mastic
Henna	Spikenard
Frankincense	Bdellium
Myrrh	Crocus

and many others.

Kyphi was burned during religious festivals; employed as medicine (it was eaten, thus accounting for the raisins, honey and wine); and, according to Plutarch, was burned to "lull to sleep, allay all anxieties, and brighten the dreams."

Many of the recipes used by the Egyptians haven't yet been translated. Others haven't been documented by ancient evidence. However, ancient Egyptian use of scented plants is intriguing. Here are some specific plants and old lore associated with them:

CINNAMON: Numerous pharaohs offered this rich inner bark to deities. It was also used in embalming.

CUMIN: (*Carum carvii*) A form of this common herb was known as *ami*. Pliny states that Egyptian women smelled the spice during sexual intercourse to ensure conception. Rameses III offered 5 *heket* (a measure) of cumin to Ra at Heliopolis.

MARJORAM: Mummies were decorated with this fragrant plant.

MYRRH: A much-offered incense, myrrh was also one of the spices used to pack body cavities during embalming.

SAFFLOWER (*Carthamus tinctorius*): The Egyptians may have worn this flower during religious and secular festivals. It was also used for mummy decoration.

WATER LILY: (*Nymphaea coerula*) Long erroneously called "lotus," this was a symbol of the Sun. Associated with Ra, Hapi, Atum, Horus and many other deities, the delicious fragrance of the blue and yellow flowers was firmly linked with Egyptian religion. The flower heads were also soaked in wine to create an intoxicating beverage which was drunk at feasts and festivals.

THE SUMERIANS AND BABYLONIANS

It is difficult to separate the practices of these two distinct cultures, for the Sumerians had a great influence on the Babylonians, who recorded much of the literature of their forebears in the Sumerian language.

However, we know that both of these peoples, who lived in the fertile crescent, used incense. The Sumerians may have even been fuming juniper berries to the goddess Inanna before the Egyptians practiced organized religion. Later, the Babylonians continued the ritual by burning the sweet perfume on Ishtar's altars.

Juniper seems to have been the commonest incense but other plants were used. Cedarwood, pine, cypress, myrtle, calamus and many others were fumed and offered to the deities. Frankincense and myrrh, apparently unknown in the days of Sumer, were used by the later Babylonians. Herodotus records that 1,000 talents of frankincense were smouldered during a single religious festival in Babylon.

Collections of magical rituals from these times have survived. These clay tablets show that the Sumerians and Babylonians lived in a world of deities, spirits and ghosts. Some of these could be harmful to humans and were believed to cause illness.

Priests performed incantations to exorcise these disease-bearing spirits from the body to cure their patients. Such operations were usually accompanied by the burning of incense. The censer (incense burner), an important part of Sumerian and Babylonian healing magic, was often placed at the head of the sick person's bed.

The *baru* was a Babylonian priest expert in the art of divination. One technique used incense: cedar shavings were thrown onto the incense burner. The direction in which the smoke rose was thought to determine the future. If the smoke moved to the right, victory or success was the answer. If to the left, defeat.

THE GREEKS AND ROMANS

The Greeks believed that scented plants sprang from the goddesses and gods who were thus pleased by the fragrances dedicated to their use. Many of their ritual uses of aromatic plants closely resemble those of the Egyptians: they anointed the deceased, burned incense on altars and lavished expensive scent on their bodies.

The Greeks believed that the fresh scents rising from living plants maintained physical health. Their houses were constructed with rooms that opened onto herb and flower gardens.

Perhaps the best-known use of odorous plants among the Greeks was the practice of crowning Olympic victory with chaplets of heavily scented laurel (bay) leaves.

Roses, carnations, lilies, myrtle, cardamom, iris, marjoram, spikenard, even quinces and pomegranates were all used for their scents.

A celebrated Greek perfumer, Megalus, invented a scent known as Megaleion. To make it, cinnamon, myrrh and burnt (charred?) frankincense were soaked in oil of balanos. Scented oils such as these were also made with olive oil. Wine-based perfumes were popular and rose was added to nearly every mixture.

The Greeks anointed their heads with perfumed unguents, especially those of roses, to prevent intoxication. Apple blossom, iris or spikenard-scented unguents were used for the same purpose.

Additionally, the Greeks inhaled specific perfumes to heal inner ailments. Oils scented with quince or white violet eased stomach upset. Grape-leaf perfume was used to clear the head. Garlands of roses were worn to relieve headache.

The Greeks burned incense during funeral ceremonies and honored the dead by placing fragrant
flowers on graves and tombs. This latter custom seems
to have been in use since the earliest times, for the
scents of flowers, with their close association with
divinity, were fitting objects to place with deceased
persons, with prayers and hopes that the goddesses
and gods would wrap them in Their loving embraces
after physical life had ended.

When Greece fell to Rome, the conquerors learned
much about perfume from the conquered. The Romans
carried the use of perfumes to such an extravagent
extent that even scented earthenware cups were popular. These were created by soaking the cups with perfume prior to use.

Such vast quantities of scented plant materials
were consumed by the populace for personal perfuming that in 565 a law was passed which forbade the use
of exotic scents by private citizens. This extraordinary
action seems to have been prompted by the fear that
there wouldn't be sufficient incense to burn on the
altars of the deities.

In the Roman document containing this law, the
following scents are specified as suitable to specific
deities: costus to Saturn; cassia and benzoin to Jove;
ambergris to Venus. Laurel and savin were recommended for invoking nearly every deity.

All this incense-burning in these cultures de-
scended from the ancient practice of leaving bunches
of wild flowers and herbs at small rural shrines.

AMERICAN INDIANS

The native peoples of the Americas lived in harmony with the Earth, reverencing it as the source of all life. Through centuries of trial and error, they achieved an understanding of the uses of wild plants which later settlers will ever equal.

These peoples used plant materials for food; cording; medicine; to create brooms and other domestic tools; as clothing and for bodily decoration (including charcoal for tattooing); for shelter; for children's toys such as dolls and for ritual purposes, including sacred poles, rattles, prayer sticks and charms.

All this is fairly well known. What isn't common knowledge is that various tribes of American Indians also practiced a form of magical aromatherapy, using the scents of certain plants for specific purposes.

These peoples must have been fascinated by the shapes, color and textures of the plants that grew around them. Those that possessed intense scents in their natural states or when burned probably generated more interest and, therefore, experimentation into ritual methods of use.

Their reverence for the Earth and its myriad life forms led these peoples to discover that plants contained energies. Scented plants in particular were used for magical purposes.

Here are some of those perfumed plants and their ritual uses among various Indian tribes, collected in the early part of this century from living individuals:*

---

* Gilmore, Melvin R., *Uses of Plants by the Indians of the Missouri River Region* and Murphey, Edith Van Allen, *Indian Uses of Native Plants*. See Bibliography for publication information.

BLOODROOT (*Sanguinaria canadensis*): This root was rubbed into the palm by Ponca bachelors desirous of marriage. If the man succeded in touching his scented hand to the object of his desire, marriage was thought to follow within five or six days.

BUSH MORNING-GLORY (*Ipomoea lepthophylla*): The Pawnee burned the root of this plant to halt nightmares.

CEDAR (*Juniperus virgiania*). One source of cedarwood oil, this fragrant tree was much used by Plains Indians. Cedar twigs were placed on hot stones in sweat lodges for purification. The Pawnee burned twigs of this tree, much like the bush morning-glory, to banish nightmares and nervous conditions.

COLUMBINE, WILD: (*Aquilegia canadensis*). Unmarried men among the Omaha and Ponca crushed the seeds of this plant and rubbed the resulting powder between the palms, which scented them with a pleasant perfume. Simply touching a young woman was sufficient to captivate her by the power of the fragrance.

FRAGRANT BEDSTRAW (*Galium triflorum*): Those who feel the last usage was chauvinistic will like this one. Omaha women used fragrant bedstraw as a perfume, for as it withers it gives off a delicate odor similar to that of sweetgrass (see below). It was worn, probably as perfume is worn today, to attract or to keep mates.

FUZZY-WEED (*Artemesia dracunculoides*) The Winnebago tribe placed the chewed root of this plant on clothing to attract love and to secure good hunting. The effect, in either case, depended on getting upwind of the desired object (person or animal) and allowing the breeze to carry the scent of the plant to them. If it was combined with mental pictures of the desired outcome, this was the purest form of magical aromatherapy.

PRICKLY ASH (*Zanthoxylum americanum*): Young men of the Omaha used the fruits of this shrub as a love-perfume to attract women.

SAGE, WILD: This isn't a true sage but consists of various species of the mugwort family (*Artemesia*). Wild sage was burned to purify an area of negative energies by many tribes, especially the Omaha and Ponca. Known as Wachanga to the Dakota, it may have played a role in the famous sun dance.

Various species of "sage," recognized by their distinct appearances, were used for different purposes. The Omaha, Pawnee, Dakota, Winnebago and many other groups used sage for purification, bathing with the plant if they'd broken a tribal law or unwittingly touched a sacred object. It was also burned to release its purifying energies within the scented smoke.

The highly fragrant, silvery-white plants were known to contain energy which protected against negative powers, and so were often used for purification at the start of ceremonies of all kinds. See Fuzzy-Weed above for more wild sage uses.

SWEETGRASS (*Hierochloe odorata*), is a narrow-leaved plant of the American plains. Among some tribes, the dried grass was plaited into a thick braid, the end of which was ignited during ceremonies to invoke the presence of beneficial deities. This practice is being rediscovered by both Indians and non-Indians alike and is used in contemporary "smudging" rituals, wherein the smoke from burning sweetgrass, sage and/or other plants is used to purify individuals prior to spiritual rituals.

Sweetgrass, which has a vanilla-like fragrance when burned, was also added to mixtures smoked during pipe ceremonies to summon good powers.

YELLOW EVENING PRIMROSE (*Oenothera hookeri*). The root of this attractive plant was used as a hunting charm. Rubbed onto moccasins and the hunter's body, it attracted deer and avoided encounters with snakes. (Snake bite was one of the commonest medical conditions among some American Indian tribes.)

THE ANCIENT HAWAIIANS

If you've been to Hawaii, you may have been enchanted by the fragrances of hundreds of tropical flowers. Most of these (including plumeria, gardenia, tuberose, carnation, virtually every species of orchid and many others) were brought by Europeans or Asian centuries after the first settlers landed on the shores of Hawaii between 500 and 1,000 C.E.

However, the ancient Hawaiians found scented plants on these high volcanic islands when they arrived, and brought others with them from their home, currently believed to have been the Society Islands. When they had established their civilization, which was later absorbed into a new migration in around 1500 C.E., perfumes were widely used by the peoples for ritual and secular purposes.

To ward off the effects of countless hours of swimming in the ocean, they anointed their hair and bodies with scented coconut oil. The grated meat of the coconut, along with odoriferous plants such as *maile* (see discussion below), were placed in dried gourds in full sunlight. Water was poured over this.

Solar heat caused the plant's essential oils—as well as the oil in the coconut—to separate and mingle on top of the water. This was strained and used as a fragrant skin softener.

The Hawaiians had many other non-ritual uses of fragrant plants, such as scenting *kapa* (the bark cloth used for bedding and clothing), and using wild ginger (*awapuhi*) juice during massage. They were reknowned for their skill at massage, and their use of scented oils seems to point to an early form of conventional aromatherapy.

Leis were first created from shells and feathers. Later, fragrant leaves and flowers were used in fashioning these offerings to Hawaiian deities. Laka, the goddess of the hula, is still given leis. In pre-missionary days, the leis around the dancers' necks belonged to the Goddess.

MAILE (*Alyxia olivaeformis*), a twining, shiny leafed vine that grows in Hawaiian rain forests, was and still is considered to be a sacred plant. Its warm, enchanting fragrance is released by bruising the stems and leaves, and increases in power as the plant dries. *Maile* was placed on every altar built for Laka.

An interesting example of the divine aspects of this plant is the idea that, if you can smell *maile* somewhere in Hawaii but can't see the plant, nearby lies an ancient temple dedicated to the goddesses and gods of old Hawaii.

HALA (*Pandanus odoratissimus*), a common Polynesian plant, was also used in perfume magic in old Hawaii. The smell of the male blossom was thought to arouse sexual desires, and so women, in earlier times, used the fragrance of these flower clusters to excite men. Subtler uses included the fragrancing of oils and clothing with *hala* pollen for aphrodisiac purposes.

PUKIAWE (*Styphelia Tameiameiae*), found in higher elevations on these volcanic islands, was of vital use in earlier times. Before the collapse of the *kapu* (taboo) system in 1819, chiefs couldn't mingle with commoners without breaking serious *kapu*, many of which would have sent the commoners to their deaths at the hands of the official executioners.

However, a chief could temporarily break this taboo by enclosing himself (or herself) in a small hut. A *kahuna* burned *pukiawe* in the hut and the smoke from the plant plus the prayers chanted while it fumed, lifted the *kapu*. This is one of the few instances I've been able to find of Hawaiian incense use.

IN SUMMARY

Peoples all over the world, including Africa, Asia Europe, Australia, South America, the Pacific Islands and those areas discussed above, have used the powers of fragrant plants to produce specific changes in their lives.

These changes included inducing spiritual connection with Deity; drawing love or mates; heightening sexual arousal; purifying the body prior to ritual; healing the sick and guarding against negative energies.

Magical aromatherapy, in one form or another, has been with us from the earliest great civilizations. It is as old as the moment when a human being first smelled the delicious scent rising from a flower and recognized it as pure energy springing from all-mighty Mother Nature.

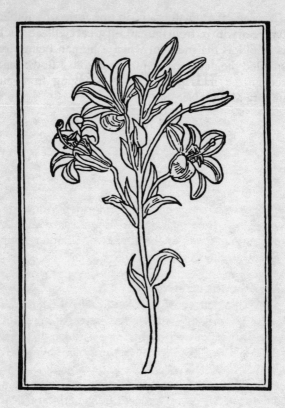

CHAPTER THREE

FRAGRANT
PLANT MATERIALS

Magical aromatherapy utilizes three forms of aromatics: fresh plants, dried plant materials and essential oils. This chapter looks at the first two. Chapter Four examines true essential oils.

Fresh Aromatic Plants

Fresh plants contain vast amounts of energy. A small bush, vibrant with blooms, releases bursts of scented power into its surroundings. So too do twigs and leaves and bunches of flowers that have been collected from it.

Because no essential oils have evaporated from them during the drying process, fresh herbs are ideal for many types of magical aromatherapy. Those flowers that lose their scents when dry must be used fresh or in essential oil form.

Most of these plants can be grown at home in small gardens or containers. This is an excellent way to ensure a steady supply of fresh magical aromatherapy tools. If winters are cold in your area, consider growing some plants in pots which can be moved indoors until danger of frost has passed. Check your local nursery or see Appendix II for sources of seeds and starter plants.

Here are some plants you may wish to grow. All of them are best used in a fresh state (though some can be used dried—for more information concerning specific plants, see PART II). Those asterisked (*) should be used fresh. Those marked with two asterisks(**) should only be used fresh or in essential oil form.

> *Apple (the flowers)
> Basil (leaves)
> Bay (leaves)
> *Bergamot Mint (leaves)
> *Broom (flowers)
> *Calendula (flowers)
> Camomile (flowers)
> *Carnation (flowers)
> Catnip (leaves)
> *Cereus, night-blooming (flowers)
> Costmary (leaves)
> *Daffodil (flowers)
> Dill (fruit "seeds," leaves)
> Eucalyptus (leaves, seed pods)
> Fennel (fruit "seeds")
> *Freesia (flowers)
> *Gardenia (flowers)
> *Garlic (cloves, flowers)
> **Geranium (leaves)
> **Ginger (root)
> *Ginger, White (flowers)
> *Honeysuckle (flowers)

Hops (flowers)
*Hyacinth (flowers)
*Hyssop (leaves)
**Jasmine (flowers)
Lavender (flowers)
*Lemon (rind of fruit)
*Lemon Balm (leaves)
Lemongrass (leaves)
**Lemon Verbena (leaves)
*Lilac (flowers)
*Lily (flowers)
*Lily of the Valley (flowers)
**Lime (rind of fruit)
*Magnolia (flowers)
*Marjoram (leaves)
Meadowsweet (leaves)
*Melon (fruit)
*Mimosa (flowers)
*Mugwort (leaves)
*Narcissus (flowers)
*Nasturtium (flowers)
*Onion (bulb)
*Orange (rind of fruit)
*Parsley (leaves)
Pennyroyal (leaves)
Peppermint (leaves)
*Pine (needles)
*Plumeria (flowers)
**Rose (flowers)
Rosemary (leaves)
*Rue (leaves)
Sage (leaves)
*Spearmint (leaves)

*Spider Lily (flowers)
*Stephanotis (flowers)
*Sweet Pea (flowers)
*Thyme (leaves)
*Tuberose (flowers)
*Tulip (flowers)
*Water Lily (flowers)
 Woodruff (leaves)
 Yarrow (flowers)

So you don't want a full-blown garden? Get a few bulbs and tend them until spring, when they burst into fragrant beauty. The narcissus, daffodil, freesia, hyacinth and tulip are easy to grow in this manner.

If you don't wish to garden, other options for obtaining fresh plants are available. Many of the flowers sold by florists are magically potent. However, some (such as roses and carnations) have been hybridized for their staying power, their appearance and color, with scent losing out to these other three factors. So many hot-house blooms have little fragrance. Check with your nose before buying.

You probably know friends who grow plants and flowers. How about the green thumb with that rose garden? Or the gourmet cook who keeps pots of basil and rosemary in the kitchen window? If the need for these herbs rises, ask for a few small sprigs. You needn't reveal your reasons for wanting them.

Do not sniff plants which have been sprayed with synthetic insecticides. If you garden, use natural methods of pest control as outlined in any good organic gardening book. Before using their herbs, ask friends if the plants are "clean." Organically-grown plants are not only best, they're practically required.

Your third option? Buy them. The following fresh fruits and herbs can often be found at grocery stores and farmer's markets (many stores around the country now carry fresh herbs in the produce department):

Basil	Orange
Dill	Parsley
Garlic	Rosemary
Ginger	Sage
Lemon	Spearmint (usually
Lime	sold as "mint")
Melon	Thyme
Onion	

his doesn't include the fresh flowers now also offered in many food stores and farm stands.

If all else fails, go to a public park or arboretum, visualize and inhale the scent of the flowers or leaves associated with your needed magical change. But don't pick them!

Dried Plant Materials

Many of the more exotic tools used in magical aromatherapy are only available in dried forms. I don't know anyone with clove trees in their backyards or sandalwood gracing their gardens. Lists of reputable mail-order dealers that sell dried aromatic herbs can be found in Appendix II.

Once again, our modern grocery stores offer a wide selection of once costly spices and herbs, usually packed in air-tight glass bottles and bearing high price tags. These are fine for use in magical aromatherapy, but check local herb shops for lower prices.

Other sources include ethnic food stores (Chinese, Indian and Middle Eastern stores offer a wide variety of rare spices and herbs) as well as Chinese medicine shops.

Those plant materials which can be used in a dried state are listed below. (Those few which must be dried, cured and/or otherwise processed before use are asterisked):

Anise	Juniper
Basil	Lavender
Bay	Lemongrass
*Black Pepper	Marjoram
Camomile	Meadowsweet
*Camphor	*Mace
Caraway	*Nutmeg
Cardamom	*Oakmoss
Catnip	*Patchouly
*Cedar	Pennyroyal
Celery seed	*Peppermint
*Cinnamon	Rosemary
*Clove	*Saffron
*Coffee	Sage
*Copal	*Sandalwood
Coriander	Spearmint
Costmary	*Star Anise
Cumin	*Tonka
Deerstongue	*Vanilla
Dill	*Vetivert
Fennel	*Wood Aloe
*Galangal	Woodruff
Hops	Yarrow
*Iris (Orris)	

Most mail-order sources for herbs are reliable. They don't sell one herb as another. Some, however, through inattention or by conscious design, sell falsely-labeled herbs.

We no longer live in the days when artificial nutmegs were carved of wood and sold as the genuine item—as they were 400 years ago when they were as valuable as diamonds. Still, it pays to purchase herbs carefully.

The scented treasures of the ages, from far-flung countries scattered across the globe, can be yours for a few dollars. Dried herbs are an important part of magical aromatherapy and are as valuable in this practice as are fresh plant materials and essential oils.

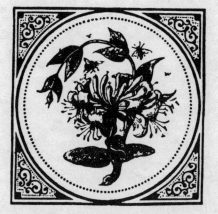

CHAPTER FOUR

ESSENTIAL OILS

Essential oils aren't oils. They aren't greasy, are usually as light as water and quickly evaporate, none of which is true of oils. Essential oils are actually volatile, aromatic substances which naturally occur within certain plants. These are what give roses, garlic and all other scented plants their distinctive odors.

Essential oils are obtained from plant materials by a number of methods, most of which are costly, potentially explosive and best left to professionals. It is virtually impossible to create true essential oils at home.

I should make one thing quite clear: *essential oils are the distilled or expressed products of naturally aromatic plant materials.* Lavender essential oil is extracted from lavender, not from a plant which smells like lavender. Additionally, *synthetics are not essential oils.*

Great confusion exists in the popular mind regarding essential oils, and yet it is so simple. If "oil of jasmine" was produced in a laboratory by a chemist, mixing appropriate chemical constituents to reproduce the scent of the flower, it is not an essential oil.

Many distributors sell synthetic "essences" that were never formed within living plant tissues. These are cheap, easily made, and, unfortunately, make up the bulk of the ingredients in 99% of the "magical" oils sold in the United States.

In magical aromatherapy, the use of true essential oils is mandatory. Synthetics won't work. This isn't a snub in the face of technology but a simple statement regarding the limitations of synthetic "essential oils."

The real thing, produced from plant materials, contain more than the terpines, aldehydes, ketones, alcohols and other constituents which create the fragrance. Because essential oils are born of plants, they have a direct link with the Earth. This subtle energy, nourished by soil, Sun and rain, vibrates within essential oils. Since we too are of the Earth and also possess this link, we can merge the energy of true essential oils with our own to create needed change.

Essential oils are concentrated plant energies. In general, essential oils are from 50 to 100 times more concentrated than the plants from which they were taken. Therefore, essential oils are powerful reservoirs of natural energies.

True essential oils may consist of hundreds of specific ingredients (chemical constitutents). Rose essential oil, for example, contains about 500 constituents, each harmoniously existing within the essential oil. These are the ingredients which give essential oils their aromas and the ability to change our minds, bodies and emotions.

True essential oils contain the correct ingredients in the correct combinations. Most are non-toxic and are easily assimilated into the body: through the nose and lungs during inhalation, via the skin during massage and by the digestive tract when taken orally. Synthetics should not be used in any of these ways.

Additionally, there's an aesthetic quality to true essential oils that synthetics will never have. Open a jar of precious yarrow oil. The scent wraps you in its energies. It is full, almost fruity. Your body and mind welcome its presence. There are no harsh, ragged edges to disturb you.

Synthetics, on the other hand, have no link with the Earth. In a magical sense, they're dead. To create them, scientists mix together only those ingredients necessary to approximate the scent of the true essential oil. The results are often hideous parodies of the real thing.

Comparing true rose essential oil (produced by steam distillation) with a synthetic rose oil is a good lesson in the importance of utilizing the genuine product. Artificial rose is sickly sweet, antiseptic and easily produces headaches. True rose essential smells like an evocative field of flowers contained within a bottle. It hums with soothing, peaceful energies. It is alive.

Genuine essential oils are usually sold in millimeter amounts and vary in price from inexpensive to costly. Nine or ten ml. bottles of the commonest essential oils (lemon, rosemary, bergamot) sell for under ten dollars. The most expensive essential oils (rose, neroli, yarrow and jasmine) are often sold in one or two ml. amounts and are usually priced at $50 and up. To give you an idea of these amounts (since the metric system has never caught on in the U.S.), the table below shows the *approximate* correspondences of milliliters to ounces:

> 1 milliliter = 1/30 ounce
> 2 milliliters = 1/16 ounce
> 4 milliliters = 1/8 ounce
> 10 milliliters = 1/3 ounce
> 15 milliliters = 1/2 ounce

Though many true essential oils are expensive, they're used in such small proportions that the overall costs are actually minimal. Essential oils are so concentrated that one drop on a cotton ball is often all that is necessary for an effective magical aromatherapy ritual (see Chapter 5 for methods of using essential oils).

It's difficult to determine whether an essential oil is genuine. One yardstick is price. I've included a chart of the general retail price ranges of true essential oils at the end of this chapter. A $3.00 price tag on "Jasmine" oil is a sure sign that it is the product of laboratories and not the Earth.

The real test is the smell. Most of us haven't been exposed to true essential oils all our lives, but it doesn't take long to build up a group of recognizable fragrances. With practice, we quickly gain the ability to identify genuine essential oils. Even the uneducated nose usually bristles at cheap imitations of the real thing.

Where do you get them? Reliable mail-order suppliers of true essential oils are listed in Appendix I of this book.

Once you've purchased a few, guard them carefully. Essential oils rapidly break down if not properly stored. Their enemies are as follows:

Light. Keep essential oils (which are always sold in dark-glassed bottles) out of sunlight.

Heat. Never place essential oils near heaters, stoves, fireplaces, lit candles or other sources of heat.

Air. Keep them firmly capped and never leave the cap off a bottle for more than a few seconds.

Moisture. The bathroom is the worst place to store essential oils. Keep them in a cool, dry place and they should last for some time.

Opinions differ, but most essential oils should continue to be effective for one to three years.

Essential oils are usually sold in small bottles with a single drop dispenser, which regulates the amount of oil used. This saves spills.

Remember: these are highly concentrated plant essences. Never drink them. Watch for allergic reactions if you're prone to these (see "Hazardous Essential Oils" in Part III of this book), and ensure that pets and children don't have access to them.

True essential oils are vital to the practice of conventional, holistic aromatherapy. In magical aromatherapy they're welcomed adjuncts to the scented plants from which they're produced. In the depths of winter, when every rosemary plant is covered with snow, we can open a bottle of the essential oil and reap the benefits of its scent.

Some of the least expensive essential oils are captured from flowers and plants which grow thousands of miles away. We can't collect ylang-ylang flowers to help us in finding love, but the essential oil is widely available. This points to another benefit from the use of essential oils: their accessibility.

If you've never experienced a true essential oil,

by all means order a few. You may be surprised at the power and energy contained in those little, brown glass bottles.

Comparative Chart of Essential Oil Prices

key: * =   under $10 per 10 milliliter bottle
** = $10 to $20 per 10 milliliter bottle
*** = $20 to $30 per 10 milliliter bottle
**** = $30 to $50 per 10 milliliter bottle
***** =   over $50 per 2 milliliter bottle
****** =   extremely expensive

NOTE: retail price ranges are averaged from current catalogs of major U.S. essential oil distributors. Actual retail prices fluctuate according to the market, availability and other factors. Names commonly used in aromatherapy for certain essential oils are included in parentheses.

BENZOIN *
BERGAMOT *
BLACK PEPPER **
CAMOMILE, GERMAN ***
CAMOMILE, ROMAN **
CAMPHOR, WHITE *
CARDAMOM ****
CEDARWOOD, ATLAS *
CEDARWOOD, VIRGINIAN *
CLARY SAGE **
CLOVE *
CORIANDER *
CYPRESS **
EUCALYPTUS *

FENNEL *
FRANKINCENSE **
GERANIUM *
GINGER*
JASMINE ABSOLUTE ****** (2 ml., *****)
JASMINE ENFLEURAGE ****** (2 ml., *****)
JUNIPER BERRY **
LAVENDER *
LEMON *
LEMON BALM (MELISSA) ******
LEMONGRASS *
LEMON VERBENA (VERBENA) ***
MARJORAM, FRENCH **
MYRRH ***
NIAOULI *
ORANGE *
NEROLI (ORANGE BLOSSOM) ****** (2 ml., ***)
PALMAROSA *
PATCHOULY *
PEPPERMINT *
PETITGRAIN *
PINE *
ROSE ABSOLUTE ***** (2 ml., ****)
ROSE OTTO ****** (2 ml., *****)
ROSEMARY *
SAGE *
SANDALWOOD **
THYME *
VETIVERT *
YARROW *****
YLANG-YLANG **

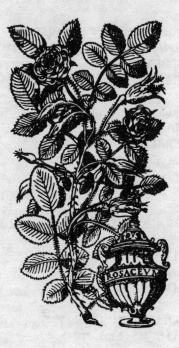

ROSACEVM

CHAPTER FIVE

METHODS AND TECHNIQUES

In its essence, magical aromatherapy is the process of visualization, inhalation of the scent of an essential oil or a plant, and the programming of personal energy. This chapter will explore the art of visualization as well as various methods of inhaling the aromas. Let's start at the beginning.

INHALATION TECHNIQUES

Several methods are available for use, and most depend upon the form of the aromatic plant materials: fresh flowers; fresh leaves; dried flowers, leaves, seeds and wood; essential oils.

Fresh Flowers

These may be purchased or harvested. If you gather your own, do so with love. Don't thoughtlessly rip off the flowers or gleefully slice cold steel through their stalks. Remember: plants are children of the Earth. They possess the same type of energy that empowers our bodies. Plants are, in a sense, our cousins, so collect them with awareness of their sacrifice. Cut gently. If you wish, leave an offering to the parent plant of a semi-precious stone or a coin.

Place the flowers in fresh water. It's best to collect heavily fragrant flowers just before sunrise when their essential oil content is at its peak. Some flowers, such as true jasmine and tuberose, release higher amounts of perfume at night. This may be the best time to collect and use them.

If you'll be performing the same ritual with these flowers for several days, replace them with fresh blossoms as they wither (preferably burying the spent ones).

Collection of the flowers isn't even necessary. If they grow in a private place, simply kneel or sit beside them and do the short ritual.

Fresh Leaves

The leaves of some plants, such as basil and rosemary, are best used in a fresh state. For these, collect according to the method described above and place in fresh water.

Dried Flowers, Leaves, Seed and Wood

No collection is necessary, but simple processing may be required before they fully release their scents. For spices such as cloves and cardamom, lightly crush in a mortar and pestle or between two rocks (place the bottom rock on a piece of paper to catch spills).

For leaves and flowers, rub between your fingers (wash hands first) to break them up.

Most woods, such as cedar and sandalwood, release so much fragrance that they needn't be ground. If this isn't the case, rub on a sharp grater for a few seconds.

Whatever method is used, only a small amount (no more than a teaspoon or so of the powdered or rubbed substance) is necessary for magical aromatherapy. If it has a sharp, strong scent, you've processed enough.

Essential Oils

The easiest method is to open the bottle and inhale, but this can lead to expensive spills (such as $50 worth of jasmine essential oil on your carpet) and certainly hastens evaporation of the costly treasures. Here are some accepted ways:

a. Place one, two or three drops of the essential oil onto a small cotton ball (not a synthetic cosmetic puff!). This should be sufficient for your purposes. For extremely costly essential oils such as rose, jasmine, yarrow and neroli, a single drop will do. Why? These are powerfully fragrant. Additionally, a two-milliliter bottle of jasmine absolute currently sells for around $50 a bottle. At two or three dollars a drop you don't want to waste it. After fragrancing the cotton ball, hold it up to your nose.

b. If you're out of cotton balls, a clean, freshly-washed handkerchief can be used. Simply place a few drops of the essential oil onto the center of the handkerchief. Don't use a handkerchief that was washed in a heavily perfumed commercial laundry soap. Buy some unperfumed castile soap and hand wash it. Hold the scented portion of the handkerchief up to your nose during the ritual.

c. Many companies (see Appendix I) sell electric essential oil diffusors. These are small appliances which automatically spread the scent and energies of an essential oil through the air. Because the essential oil isn't exposed to heat, none of its properties are destroyed or altered.

Diffusors are useful for specific rituals or to spread the energies of an essential oil throughout your home; an excellent idea for protection, love, health and purification.

To use, simply place a few drops of the essential oil in the glass "nebulizer" and let it do its work.

d. Potpourri simmerers (those two-part ceramic items) also diffuse essentials oils through the air. The heat necessary to accomplish this purpose may alter the oil but, generally speaking, satisfactory results will be obtained.

Add about a half cup of water to the top portion, light the small candle which sits in the bottom half, set the top over it and place a few drops of the essential oil into the water. As the water simmers, it will spread the fragrance. Sit or stand beside the simmerer and inhale the scent as you visualize. As with diffusors, potpourri simmerers will spread the essential oil's aroma (and, therefore, its energies) over a wide area.

Heavy oils with slow evaporation rates (such as sandalwood and patchouly) don't work well in potpourri simmerers, but most others perform well.

e. Bring distilled or purified water to a boil in a nonmetallic pot. Place this in a large, heat-proof bowl and add a few drops of the essential oil. Inhale the scented, energized steam as you visualize.

f. A few essential oils listed in this book can be used in baths. However, don't experiment by adding strange essential oils to your bathwater. Some are highly irritating to the mucous membranes and the skin in general. The last effect you want from a magical bath is an itchy, burning sensation. Always avoid citrus oils (orange, petitgrain, lemongrass, lemon verbena, lemon balm) and strong spices (clove, cinnamon, nutmeg).

A half-tub or less of water is fine. Add the essential oil to the bath drop by drop just before you get in, so that it doesn't evaporate from the water's heat. For most baths, six to ten drops is plenty.

Relax. Visualize.

VISUALIZATION

This is a simple, natural process that most of us perform every day. An example? Imagine yourself waking up in the morning, looking at the clock, laughing and going back to sleep. That's visualization. Or, in your mind's eye, see yourself suddenly finding a 50-dollar bill in your purse or wallet. That, too, is visualization.

Visualization is the art of creating mental images. Mental dialogue (such as thinking, "Gee, wouldn't it be great if I could fall in love with someone who loves me?") isn't visualization. The word *visual* indicates that pictures, not words, are involved.

Every invention, every article of clothing we're wearing, everything that every human being has ever created, is the product of visualization. An image appeared or was formed in the maker's mind. Using hands and raw materials, the image was translated into physical reality.

In magical aromatherapy, we form a mental image of our necessary, needed change. Prosperity; love; health; protection. We paint an image with the imagination, creating a mental illustration which uniquely encapsulates the change we wish to make. Though I give specific examples in Part II of this book, here are a few to get you started.

Peace: When you're suffering from the effects of stress, are emotionally distraught or at your wit's end, *see* yourself (remember, don't recite the words describing this scene in your head) slipping into a warm, soothing stream or standing under a gentle waterfall. The water laps at your body, spirit and soul, easing tensions, unknitting your muscles, relaxing your central nervous system. See and feel peace flooding through yourself. Then inhale the fragrance which promotes this state. Continue to visualize as the aroma works its magic.

Money: When you're financially depleted, visualize yourself cashing large checks and depositing money into your bank account or stashing it in your home safe—if you have one. (Remember: don't think, "Wow! I have lots of money now!")

Love: If you need a mutually satisfying, interpersonal relationship, visualize yourself in his or her arms, enjoying quiet walks, sex and everything else you associate with love. Don't create an image of that man you saw at the office yesterday or the cute woman down the hall. Do not visualize a specific person. See yourself and another human being in a happy relationship.

Work with visualization every day and it will be increasingly easy. You may be surprised at the capabilities of your conscious mind.

ALLOWING THE CHANGE

Magical aromatherapy manifests the strongest changes when we allow ourselves to accept the new energies. If we visualize and inhale but stubbornly cling to our old mindset and ways, we're setting ourselves up for defeat.

If you've long had a negative view of love, quench those thoughts before trying a love-attracting ritual. If you're worried about the problems and responsibilities of money, transform them into an eagerness for the challenge. If you've long abused your body, virtually asking to be sick, change your habits and lifestyle before performing a health or healing ritual.

PREVENTION

This is certainly better than cure. Before you're depleted, run-down and sick, perform a simple health ritual rather than waiting to do a healing. Before you're out of money, boost up your prosperity. When you first feel tensions building to a seemingly insurmountable level, use some peaceful aromas to stave off an attack of depression. Watch yourself and your life. Be ruthless in your self-assessment, and use magical aromatherapy to prevent problems prior to their occurrence.

ON MAGICAL AROMATHERAPY

This is a simple form of magic which utilizes the energies resident within natural, organic scents and those of our minds and bodies. It is *not* a supernatural practice. Every process at work within magical aromatherapy hasn't been fully explained yet but that doesn't invalidate it.

What could be more natural than ourselves and the fragrant plants around us?

ALLERGIC REACTIONS

Some essential oils and fragrant plants may cause allergic reactions in some individuals. If you know you're allergic to, say, roses, don't inhale the flowers or rose essential oil at all.

If you discover that you have severe reactions to a specific scent, simply don't use it. Others are available. (See the tables in Part III for suggested substitutions.)

DANGERS

The only real dangers in magical aromatherapy are from certain essential oils. Remember, these are highly concentrated forms of plants. Sage is a common culinary seasoning, yet the oil contains the toxic substance *thujone*. Mugwort, fennel, marjoram, pennyroyal, rue and some other essential oils have been determined to be dangerous, so don't use them. Pregnant women should be especially careful with many of them. See "Hazardous Essential Oils" in Part III of this book for more information.

And remember—*never* take any essential oil internally!

LAST THOUGHTS

As stated in Chapter 1, magical aromatherapy isn't intended to treat serious illnesses or emotional states. See a qualified health practitioner to treat these problems. Conventional aromatherapists (those who have been fully trained to work with essential oils and massage therapy) are often incredibly successful. Their treatments can be used with good results in combination with orthodox medicine or, in some cases, in place of it. See Appendix III for sources of qualified aromatherapists.

Above all, magical aromatherapy is a valuable tool, a natural practice which touches our souls with the scented energies of the Earth. It is an age-old art only now resurfacing in these trying times, offering hope from flowers and precious essential oils.

May you use it to manifest positive, needed changes in your life.

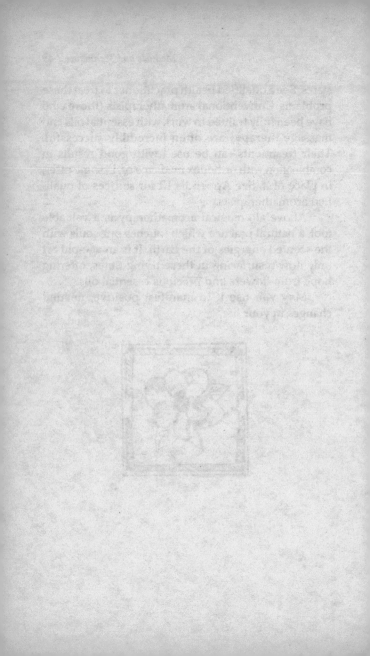

PART II

THE AROMAS

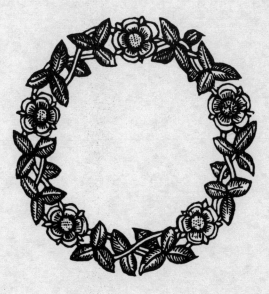

Introduction

Here are discussions of the magical properties and uses of 100 natural aromatics—fresh herbs, dried herbs and essential oils. As in previous books, I've given a fairly rigid structure to this section:

COMMON NAME: (in English)
SPECIFIC NAME: (useful for determining exactly which plant is recommended for use. Many "jasmines" are sold in nurseries, but only a few of them are true jasmines.)
AKAs: (other names by which the plant or essential oil is known)
PART USED: (essential oil, leaves, flowers; dried or fresh)
RULING PLANET:
RULING ELEMENT: (more information on the planets and elements can be found in Part III)
MAGICAL INFLUENCES: (the specific areas in which the aroma effects changes)
LORE: (some articles contain historical, ritual and magical information relating to the fragrance)

This information precedes the bulk of each article, which describes some of the magical ways in which the scent can be used. For a few fragrances, one last section follows:

Warning: (This appears only as needed. As mentioned in Chapter 5, some essential oils and fresh plants can be dangerous when unwisely used.)

Keep in mind that much of this information is personal. Where my correspondences and ritual suggestions don't link with your response to an aroma, feel free to change them.

We may have highly individual emotional responses to aromas. During a recent class that I taught on this subject, one man said that the scent of wood aloe smelled like the back of a New York taxi cab. For him, it was useless in promoting sprituality.

During another session, the aroma of neroli essential oil produced feelings of comfort and care in a woman whose mother had bathed her with neroli-scented soap.

So read the following information. Experience the scents themselves. Notice their effects, particularly in the emotional sphere. Use them accordingly.

Additionally, use only those aromas which you enjoy. It would be pointless to inhale the scent of, say, basil to manifest money in your life if you detest the odor.

Listen to your body as well. Don't use plants or essential oils which produce allergic reactions.

I've purposely avoided including rare or completely unavailable plants and essential oils in this section. All of these scents—in starter plants, essential oil or dried forms—can be easily obtained from the companies listed in Appendices I and II.

This section can be read straight through or used as reference. Some of the information contained here is collated into tables in Section III.

Welcome to my garden. Welcome to the wonders of magical aromatherapy!

APPLE
(Pyrus malus)

PART USED: fresh flowers
PLANET: Venus
ELEMENT: Water
MAGICAL INFLUENCES: Love, Peace, Happiness

When pink and white blossoms unfurl on the naked branches of apple trees, magic is soon in the air. The delicate, sweet scent of fresh apple flowers never loses its appeal—partly, perhaps, because no true essential oil is available. We can only enjoy it for a few months every year.

When I was growing up, my father planted an apple tree in the back yard. This was my introduction to this delicious scent.

If you have access to apple trees, go to them when they bloom, especially if you're depressed. Inhale the fragrance that rises from the shell-like flowers, breathing in peace, contentment and freedom from worry. Visualize the odor itself washing away all negative thoughts. Dispel these as you exhale.

This scent is also ideal for promoting thoughts of love, both for yourself as well as toward others. It seems cruel to break off a flowering branch from a tree, but a few blooms can be gathered and used until they wither. Say a prayer of thanks to the tree as you collect them and treasure the flowers. When they've dried, bury them in the Earth beneath the tree.

Any and all "apple blossom essential oils" you may see in stores are synthetic.

BASIL
(Ocimum basilicum)
PART USED: fresh leaves, dried leaves
PLANET: Mars
ELEMENT: Fire
MAGICAL INFLUENCES: Conscious mind, Happiness, Peace, Money
LORE:

Those of us who know this herb in the familiar form of pesto sauce may be surprised at the rich history behind basil. In India in past times, the deceased were buried under the floors of houses. A pot of basil was placed on a window sill and carefully tended in the name of the deceased. The spicy odor which rose from the leaves naturally perfumed the air.

Basil was regarded with suspicion upon its introduction to Europe. The story arose (which was reported by Culpeper—see Bibliography) that a man smelled basil so often that it bred a scorpion in his head. Perhaps this was actually a headache caused by an overdose of the strong scent.

In the West Indies, basil is soaked in water and the scented liquid is sprinkled around stores to attract buyers and good luck.

RITUAL USES:

Basil is used in either fresh or dried forms. The fresh leaves are fine and the plant is fun to grow. Use the dried herb if nothing else is available.

Basil has a rich, spicy scent. Most contemporary aromatherapists agree that it stimulates the conscious mind, refreshing it and reducing mental fatigue.

Because spicy scents are used to smooth decision-making, basil, with its mind-clearing properties, is ideal for this purpose. Simply crush a leaf and sniff while clearing your mind. The correct path will reveal itself.

The scent of basil is also ideal for elevating your spirits. Simply inhaling its fragrance makes it virtually impossible to remain upset or nervous. As long ago as the 16th century John Gerard wrote that "The smell of Basil . . . taketh away sorrowfulness . . . and maketh a man merry and glad." When you're next hit with the blues, call upon the energy of basil.

Basil has long been associated with money in folk magic. To attract increased money, inhale the odor and visualize your pockets bulging, your bank account accumulating a higher balance, or any other image which you associate with money.

This scent is also said to relieve headache (though it didn't for that guy with a scorpion in his brain) and stimulates the appetite.

Warning: Do not use basil essential oil internally. Recent studies indicate that basil essential oil is hazardous and potentially toxic.

BAY

(Laurus nobilis)

PART USED: essential oil, fresh or dried leaves
PLANET: the Sun
ELEMENT: Fire
MAGICAL INFLUENCES: Psychic awareness, Purification

The leaves of this European native were long used by the Greeks to crown victors, but most of us know them as a potherb. I remember finding a bay leaf in one of my mother's stews as a boy and wondering if it had blown in through the window.

The scent of bay is sharp and crisp. To promote psychic awareness in general, or as needed, crumple a fresh leaf, crush a dried leaf or put a few drops of the essential oil onto a cotton ball. Sit comfortably in a chair or on the ground. Relax your body and conscious mind. Inhale the fragrance—the same scent that the Delphic Oracle in Greece smelled. Visualize your conscious mind freeing its grip on your psychic mind. Allow the odor to permeate your being, calling forth psychic consciousness.

When you've made the connection between the two halves of your mind, discover what you need to know.

An alternate use of bay: inhale the aroma when you feel psychically dirty or simply wish to bring some positive changes to your life. Visualize its odor sweeping you clean. This is a powerful purification.

BENZOIN

(Styrax benzoin)

PART USED: essential oil

PLANET: Mercury
ELEMENT: Air
MAGICAL INFLUENCES: Physical energy, Magical
  energy, Conscious mind

This was one of the first fragrances that I worked with in my magical studies. The essential oil possesses a warm, sweet, vanilla-like odor. It is dark, thick and viscous. Unlike most other essential oils, benzoin will leave an oily mark on paper.

The essential oil is inhaled to revitalize the physical body. This is ideal in those times of great exertion when you need an extra few moments of energy.

The increased bioelectrical (physical) energy produced by inhaling benzoin essential oil can be utilized in heavy magical operations, such as the protection of a home or car. Generally speaking, any scent which energizes the physical body also produces a larger reserve of magical power.

As with basil, the scent of benzoin stimulates the conscious mind.

BERGAMOT
(Citrus bergamia)

PART USED: essential oil
PLANET: Sun
ELEMENT: Fire
MAGICAL INFLUENCES: Peace, Happiness, Restful
  sleep

Bergamot grows on the sun-drenched coast of Italy and elsewhere on the Mediterranean. It is a small fruit that yields a citrusy fragrance which Jeanne Rose described as being "yummy"—and I heartily agree.

Bergamot oil is soothing to frazzled nerves and stressed bodies. It is also uplifting to that part of us which isn't physical—to our soul, if you wish to call it that. Inhaling the aroma, even without visualization, relieves depression and the everyday tensions that are so much a part of our lives.

At night, inhale the odor to produce a restful, relaxing sleep.

True bergamot oil is a long-time ingredient in cosmetic perfumery and is often confused with bergamot mint (see next entry).

Warning: Bergamot oil should not be placed on the skin due to its capability of increasing the skin's ability to tan, which can lead to burns.

BERGAMOT MINT
(Mentha citrata)
AKA "Bergamot Orange" and "Orange Bergamot"
PART USED: fresh leaves
PLANET: Mercury
ELEMENT: Air
MAGICAL INFLUENCES: Physical energy, Prosperity

A crisp, citrusy scent rises from the leaves of this handsome plant. Sniff it, with visualization, to increase physical (and magical) energy. The fragrance is so refreshing that this isn't difficult to do.

To increase the flow of money into your life, to ensure that you spend wisely and take advantage of offers to earn more, inhale bergamot mint while visualizing yourself as doing just that—making the correct financial decisions, sticking to budgets, welcoming and allowing money to come into your life.

A folk magic spell directs us to rub fresh bergamot

mint leaves onto paper money before spending it to ensure its return. Inhale the scent and visualize while doing this.

BLACK PEPPER
(Piper nigrum)
AKA: "Pepper"

PART USED: dried fruits, essential oil
PLANET: Mars
ELEMENT: Fire
MAGICAL INFLUENCES: Mental alertness, Physical energy, Protection, Courage

You may be surprised to find black pepper in this book, but few will argue that it contains a powerful scent. Snorting the powdered herb will cause sneezing, but crushing a few peppercorns in a mortar and pestle—or taking a quick sniff from a bottle of the true essential oil—won't have this effect.

In fact, the essential oil, while possessing the distinctive sharpness of pepper, has an almost sweet undertone as well.

The powerful scent is useful for sharpening mental faculties and energizing the body. Also, sniff the essential oil to remain awake, particularly when driving at night.

Other, lesser-known qualities of black pepper fall strictly into the area of magic. Its protective qualities are rather effective when combined with visualization. This is one recommended method of use:

You probably won't have a bottle of the oil with you when walking down a dark street or when suddenly confronted with a potentially dangerous situation. However, you can take steps beforehand to build up your own natural self-defensive energies. These energies will repel negativity of all kinds, even that stemming from would-be assailants.

During the day, while alone, crush three or four peppercorns or place two drops of black pepper essential oil onto a cotton ball. *Strongly* visualize a whirlwind surrounding your body, a psychic force so powerful that it knocks away all incoming negative energy. Sniff the warm, protective odor as you visualize. Fuse the scent and your visualization in your conscious mind. Maintain this for 15 to 30 seconds.

Repeat once a day for a week. When danger threatens, recall the scent and the visualization.

Additionally, sniff black pepper before making an important phone call, confronting an audience or prior to any nervewracking situation. Take in the strength of black pepper to see you through rough times. It demonstrably bolsters your courage.

BROOM
(Cystisus scoparius)

PART USED: fresh flowers
PLANET: Mars
ELEMENT: Fire
MAGICAL INFLUENCES: Protection of home, Purification, Peace

Various varieties of broom can be found in nurseries. The sweet fragrance of yellow broom flowers is certainly cheering, but its magical energies are more diverse than may be imagined.

Protection: Collect the fresh flowers from the plant with thanks. Place them in a jar of water and set in the house. Sit or stand before them, inhaling the delicious aroma. Visualize your home as a guarded, secure place. Feel and see the energry from the flowers traveling into you, mixing with your own energy and then streaming out (perhaps from your outstretched fingertips) into the walls and doors to form a protective barrier around your home. Leave the flowers in the house to continue to permeate it with protective energies. Alternately, sniff them to bolster your own personal protection.

Purification: The sweet scent of the fresh flowers also purifies our thought processes, bodies and souls. You needn't cut the blooms for this purpose—simply bend down or sit on the Earth beside the short plant and smell away.

Peace: Inhale the sweet aroma of fresh broom flowers and allow it to promote calm and tranquility within yourself. Place in every room of the house to spread soothing energies.

CALENDULA
(Calendula officinalis)

PART USED: fresh flowers
PLANET: Sun
ELEMENT: Fire
MAGICAL INFLUENCES: Health, Psychic dreams, Comfort
LORE:

This flower's name stems from the Latin *calends*, the word denoting the first day of each month (and the origin of the English "calendar"). It was so called because the yellow and orange flowers were said to be in bloom on every calends throughout the year in ancient Rome.

MAGICAL USES:

I've called this flower by its true name rather than the common misnomer, marigold, since the calendula is often confused with the Mexican flower *Tagetes* spp. There is a resemblance, but the two flowers have vastly different energies.

This plant, prized in medicinal herbalism, also has magical aromatherapy applications. The scent of the flowers strengthens and maintains health. At one time in the past, fresh calendula blossoms were sniffed to sharpen the eyesight. This was probably pure sympathetic magic, for the flowers resemble eyes.

Sniff the aroma of calendula at night just before going to bed to produce psychic dreams.

For centuries, the blooms have been sniffed to comfort the weary and distressed.

CAMOMILE
(Anthemis nobilis)
(Anthemis mixta)
German Camomile: *Matricaria chamomilla*
AKA: "Chamomile"

PART USED: fresh or dried flowers, essential oil
PLANET: Venus
ELEMENT: Water
MAGICAL INFLUENCES: Sleep, Meditation, Peace

Our word "camomile" stems from the Greek *chamaimelon*, or "earth apple," an adequate description of the flower's scent.

I've listed three distinct varieties of this plant above. All are used in magical aromatherapy. *Anthemis nobilis* (known as Roman Camomile) is well known for its use in Europe and the U.S. as a sedative tea. Any type can be used for the purposes discussed below with equal effectiveness.

At night, sniff the essential oil, fresh or dried camomile flowers to induce sleep. Or, during the day, invite these energies into yourself to promote peace and to remove the effects of stress and tension.

Many people meditate every day. If you sometimes have trouble slipping into the proper state, smell camomile to reduce tension and to facilitate meditation.

The essential oils of *Anthemis nobilis* and *Anthemis mixta* are yellowish. The essential oil of *Matricaria chamomilla*, German Camomile, is a beautiful shade of blue. The substance responsible for this color, azulene, isn't present within the plant itself but naturally forms during the extraction process which creates the oil. Just gazing at it is relaxing. Combined with the delicious scent, the oil works wonders in soothing stressed persons.

All are rather expensive. However, if you can only afford to buy a few essential oils, camomile should be one of the first ones you purchase (see Appendix I: Suppliers).

I can't resist adding that the fragrance of Roman Camomile essential oil, which is sweet and fruity and quite delicious, reminds me of freshly-baked banana bread.

CAMPHOR
(Cinnamomum camphora)

PART USED: essential oil
PLANET: Moon
ELEMENT: Water

MAGICAL INFLUENCES: Purification, Physical energy, Celibacy

LORE:

Ancient camphor trees guard Taoist and Buddhist temples throughout China.

Camphor was (and still may be) an ingredient in the manufacture of firecrackers. In earlier times, small pieces of camphor were worn around the neck to guard against infectious diseases.

MAGICAL USES:

Most of us know this scent from mothballs, but these contain artificial camphor, not the genuine substance. To this day many drug stores sell small, cellophane-wrapped squares boldly marked "camphor." The fine print on these packages warns that this is synthetic camphor, and that inhaling the vapors can be hazardous to our health.

White camphor oil is much safer to use than the synthetic form. This is a powerful, cool scent which can be inhaled to speed recovery from colds. When sniffed with the proper visualization, the scent of camphor is excellent for self-purification and stimulation of the physical body.

Several hundred years ago, religious men and women systematically inhaled camphor to lessen and finally to kill all desire for sexual activity. If you wish to cool down, give camphor a sniff or two.

However, inhaling this permeating scent for more than a few seconds at a time can lead to severe headaches. So visualize, open the bottle, take a quick whiff and close it up again.

Crystalline camphor can be used in place of the essential oil but is much harder to find. I enjoy camphor—the way it looks, the way it smells. But this powerful scent should be used with respect.

If you wish to grow your own, camphor trees are available by mail (see Companion Plants in Appendix II). You won't be able to extract camphor, but the leaves and wood contain the familiar scent.

CARAWAY
(Carum carvi)

PART USED: dried fruits, essential oil
PLANET: Mercury
ELEMENT: Air
MAGICAL INFLUENCES: Conscious mind, Physical energy, Love

Rye bread smells and tastes so good because of the caraway fruits (often misnamed "seeds") that are added to the dough.

Caraway possesses a stimulating odor. Crush the seeds and inhale the scent to revitalize the physical body, perhaps visualizing the aroma as brilliant orange-yellow flames.

This fragrance is also refreshing to the conscious mind. Sniff to enhance alertness and to strengthen the memory.

To attract love, visualize yourself freely giving and receiving it as you smell the crushed fruits. Repeat this simple, short ritual several times a day—especially when worrying about your current relationship.

To smooth an ongoing relationship, smell and visualize the two of you working out problems and communicating. Lack of communication is the major cause of separations.

CARDAMOM
(Elettaria cardamom)
AKA: "Cardamon"

PART USED: dried seeds, the essential oil
PLANET: Venus
ELEMENT: Water
MAGICAL INFLUENCES: Love, Sex

Cardamom is the second-most expensive spice in common world trade today. Only saffron is costlier. At the time of this writing, fairly good quality cardamom sold for $2.50 an ounce in San Diego. Many stores don't carry it, so check with mail-order suppliers (Appendix II).

This is one of the most luxuriant, richest scents you're ever likely to encounter. Cardamom seeds bear an unfortunate resemblance to a small, legless insect, but their delicious fragrance (powerful even in a whole state) more than makes up for their rather peculiar appearance.

It is used throughout the Middle East and elsewhere to flavor and scent coffee. Part of its popularity may stem from its legendary property of arousing sexual desires. This effect is also felt (by some) when inhaling its odor.

If this is undesirable, simply visualize love as you smell the intoxicating fragrance. See yourself in an equally beneficial relationship. Create this state in your conscious mind and use the fragrance of cardamom to stir your own energies. After inhaling, send out your charged power and let it do its work.

The aroma of cardamom is also recommended to clear the conscious mind and to stimulate the appetite.

It may have other uses. When I let a friend smell a simmering potpourri I'd devised (largely scented with cardamom), she told me I should bag it and sell it as a drug. This statement from a very anti-drug woman points to the power of its fragrance.

Cardamom is closely related to ginger and has some of that particular plant's spiciness in its odor. The essential oil perfectly captures its fragrance and yet, somehow, lifts and heightens it in some unexplainable way. This is one of my favorite scents (is it obvious?).

CARNATION
(Dianthus carophyllus)

PART USED: fresh flowers
PLANET: Sun
ELEMENT: Fire
MAGICAL INFLUENCES: Physical energy, Magical energy, Love, Health

The name for this plant, Dianthus, means "flower of god" or "flower of Zeus." It has been in use since at least the 4th century C.E. (Common Era; the non-religious equivalent of A.D.)

Here in Southern California we're swamped with carnations. Raised in hothouses stretched along the Pacific coastline and grown across the border in Mexico, they pop up everywhere and are available all year at fairly reasonable prices.

However, the vast majority of these flowers are useless for magical aromatherapy. As has been the case with the rose, carnations have been hybridized to produce the biggest bloom size, longest stems and brightest colors. The scent has been forgotten. Thus, most carnations obtained from florist shops are virtually scentless. The red ones are an exception, but even here the spiciness is slight. Genuine carnation absolute isn't currently available.

So what can you do if you wish to utilize the intriguing energies within carnations? Get yourself some starter plants and grow your own. What better way to ensure that you have a steady supply of these fabulous blooms? Look for short-stemmed red varieties with the heaviest fragrances.

Before a potentially exhausting magical act, inhale the rich aroma of fresh carnation flowers. Accept the flower's energy into yourself. Add it to your physical store of power which will soon be released from the body during magic.

When you're suffering through a cold or some other minor illness, keep carnations around your sickbed. Inhale their odor while visualizing yourself in a healthy, healed state. If friends wish to give you flowers, you can always ask for carnations—even commercially grown ones.

These flowers, which Gerard said have an "excellent sweet smell," are also smelled, with proper visualization, to bring a spicy love into your life.

CATNIP
(Nepeta cataria)

PART USED: fresh and dried leaves
PLANET: Venus
ELEMENT: Water
MAGICAL INFLUENCES: Peace, Beauty

Rats are supposed to detest the odor of catnip.

Catnip is well known to anyone who has ever treated a feline to a bit of the herb. Its odor is penetrating and rather peculiar, and is strongest in the fresh leaves. It seems to intoxicate cats but, taken internally, has a sedative effect upon human beings.

Sniff the aroma of catnip to promote peace and happiness, especially after some trying experience.

To enhance inner and outer beauty, take a few fresh catnip leaves to a mirror. Stand before it, gazing into the reflection of your eyes. With the palette of your mind, alter your appearance in whatever manner most pleases you. When you have this visualization firmly in mind (with your eyes open, still staring at your reflection), inhale the odor of catnip at least three times. Upon each inhalation sharpen your vision.

Repeat once every three days.

CEDAR
Atlas: *Cedrus atlantica*
Red Cedar: *Juniperus virginiana*
AKA: "Cedarwood"
PART USED: dried wood, essential oil
PLANET: Sun
ELEMENT: Fire
MAGICAL INFLUENCES: Spirituality, Self-control
LORE:

In the ancient world, cedar from Lebanon was highly prized—so much so that only a few trees remain standing in that country. The name Lebanon is derived from the Akkadian word *lubbunu*, incense.

This was one of the most widely used incenses in the general Mesopotamian region and by the pre-contact American Indian tribes.

RITUAL USES:

There are few among us who aren't familiar with the rich scent of cedar. Shavings of the wood are sold in pet supply stores. The characteristic smell of pencils stems from the red cedarwood used to produce them. And many of us have at least smelled a cedarwood chest. These are ideal for storing magical supplies (everything, that is, except herbs and essential oils).

Two main cedarwood essential oils are available. Because the essential oils share similar constituents, Atlas Cedarwood (*Cedrus atlantica*) or Red Cedarwood (*Juniperus virginiana*) can be used with equal effectiveness in magical aromatherapy.

The scent of the wood and the essential oil promotes spirituality. Inhale this sweetly antiseptic, calming fragrance before religious rituals to deepen your connection with Deity.

Its spiritual qualities make the fragrance of cedar ideal for bringing ourselves into balance. Smell the aroma and visualize yourself as poised, calm, in control of your own life.

Warning: Cedarwood oil should not be used by pregnant women.

CELERY
(Apium graveolens)

PART USED: dried seed
PLANET: Mercury
ELEMENT: Air
MAGICAL INFLUENCES: Psychic awareness, Sleep

Most cooks know the rather peculiar odor of celery

seed, which has been compared to that of parsley.

To awaken your psychic awareness, crush about a teaspoon of the dried seeds and tie up in a piece of thin, cotton cloth. Inhale the odor and visualize your conscious mind relaxing (perhaps as a fist relaxes), allowing true communication with your psychic mind to occur.

To bring restful sleep, stuff small pillows with celery seed and lay your head on these.

CEREUS, NIGHT-BLOOMING
(Cereus grandiflorus)

PART USED: fresh flowers
PLANET: Moon
ELEMENT: Water
MAGICAL INFLUENCE: Psychic awareness

As a boy, I remember looking at the rather homely, straggly cactus for years, wondering why my father ever planted it. Then it formed buds. One night we all dragged chairs into the front yard and watched as the spear-shaped buds burst open into 12-inch flowers with delicate white petals and a center of hundreds of yellow stamens. It was an awesome sight. The scent was heavenly, but by morning the flowers had withered and died.

The appearance and fragrance of these flowers is exquisite. If you live in a warm climate, by all means grow a night-blooming cereus. In the future you'll be rewarded by the type of special effects Hollywood can only dream of producing.

The flowers freely exude a tangy vanilla-like aroma into the cool night air. If you have the opportunity to smell them, do so while visualizing complete control over your conscious mind, a control that nurtures psychic awareness.

This is truly one of the queens of the realm of flowers.

CINNAMON
(*Cinnamomum zeylanicum*)
Chinese Cinnamon: *Cinnamomum cassia*

PART USED: dried inner bark
PLANET: Sun
ELEMENT: Fire
MAGICAL INFLUENCES: Physical energy, Psychic awareness, Prosperity

One of the flavoring ingredients of Coca-Cola.

Slightly crush the bark to release its scent.

Inhale the warm, sweet, spicy fragrance with visualization to strengthen the physical body. The spice energizes us. This additional bioelectrical power is available for use in magical rituals.

The aroma of cinnamon also increases our ability to tap into our psychic minds. In an entirely different realm, inhale the odor of cinnamon with visualization to increase your financial base. See its rich scent oozing with money energy.

It's best to buy the "sticks" rather than the pre-ground spice, as the scent will be much stronger if you crush them in a mortar and pestle or break the sticks apart between your fingers.

Most cinnamon sold in the U.S. is actually cassia, an inferior spice with a similar fragrance and taste. Because it's all that is available to us, it will have to do.

Warning: Cinnamon essential oil is very irritating and should never be used on the skin.

CLARY SAGE
(Salvia sclarea)

PART USED: essential oil
PLANET: Mercury
ELEMENT: Air
MAGICAL INFLUENCES: Euphoria, Calm, Dreams

Clary sage is related to the common garden sage. Unlike it, though, this pink-flowered herb's essential oil is non-toxic to humans.

The essential oil has a musty, sage-like aroma. It isn't pleasing to all noses but it certainly does its work.

Perhaps clary sage's most celebrated effect upon humans is its legendary ability to induce euphoria when inhaled for a few moments. However, as Robert Tisserand warns us in his excellent book *The Art of Aromatherapy*, deliberately abusing clary sage oil for this purpose will result only in severe headache. Essential oils, like synthetic drugs, can be misused and overdoses of their scents alone are possible.

In times of great mental or emotional stress, inhale clary sage essential oil. This will allow you to temporarily release these problems. Afterward, calmly deal with them in the appropriate way.

For more general purposes, clary sage essential oil can be inhaled for short periods of time to relax the body and mind. Inhale shortly before bed to encourage sleep and to produce vivid dreams.

Marcel Lavabre, in *The Handbook of Aromatherapy*,

writes that clary sage oil may be of help in releasing female sexual dysfunction (frigidity).

Warning: Do not use clary sage in conjunction with alcohol or to excess.

CLOVE
(Syzygium aromaticum; Caryophyllus aromaticus)
PART USED: dried, unopened buds
PLANET: Jupiter
ELEMENT: Fire
MAGICAL INFLUENCES: Healing, Memory, Protection, Courage

Clove is among the most aromatic of culinary spices. Its aroma, perhaps the ultimate "spicy" fragrance, has many magical uses.

Every morning for at least a week, crush a few dried cloves while visualizing yourself as maintaining (or regaining) health. Continue to visualize as you smell the delicious aroma.

Regularly sniffing freshly ground cloves strengthens the conscious mind and, in the process, facilitates the retrieval of long-buried memories. In trying to recall "forgotten" information, inhale and visualize yourself remembering it. The aroma is also excellent for strengthening your ability to memorize new data.

Because of its pervasive odor, clove can also be used to boost our built-in protective systems utilizing a ritual such as the one outlined for black pepper above.

To heighten courage, sniff the fragrance and symbolically face the enemy. Do this *with visualization*, seeing yourself as calm and ready to take on the world (or at least that part of it which is bothering you).

Warning: Clove essential oil, whether distilled from leaf, bud or stem, is irritating to the skin and should not be used.

COFFEE
(Coffea arabica)
PART USED: the roasted seeds
PLANET: Mars
ELEMENT: Fire
MAGICAL INFLUENCES: Conscious mind, Breaking deadlocks

Who among us doesn't have strong associations with the scent of freshly brewed coffee? Even those who never drink it have certainly smelled it—in restaurants, when visiting friends, in offices, at social gatherings.

Smell the scent of the roasted, ground seeds (called beans) or brewed coffee to stimulate the conscious mind. You needn't drink it; simply savor its fragrance.

If you're faced with two decisions and are gaining no ground in deciding which course to take, calm yourself. Visualize yourself standing in the woods at the fork of a road, with two paths stretching out on either side of you. Smell the rich aroma of coffee and you will know which path to take.

COPAL
(Bursera spp.)
PART USED: gum-resin
PLANET: Sun

ELEMENT: Fire
MAGICAL INFLUENCES: Purification
LORE:

Used by the Maya, the Aztecs and many other peoples of Central and North America, copal is currently gaining in popularity as an incense for spiritual purposes.

The Otomi, a people living in Mexico, still use the smoke from smouldering copal to purify magical images designed to heal the sick. Copal is also burned in Mexican households for purification and protection.

Curiously enough, true fossilized copal (copal amber) is occasionally found.

MAGICAL USES:

As far as I know, copal isn't currently available as an essential oil. The gum-resin can be found in many U.S. shops, though the majority of this is plantation-grown in the Philippines. Little or no Mexican copal hits United States markets.

Copal best releases its rich scent when smouldered on charcoal blocks, but I couldn't do a book of this kind without mentioning it. The powdered and chunk forms emit an odor akin to frankincense but with a lighter, citrusy tone. It is a clean, crisp fragrance which is ideal for self-purification rituals.

The next time you're feeling depressed or guilty over some trifling matter, or at any other time you feel the need, smell the fragrance of copal. Visualize it pouring into you like a tiny, friendly series of whirlwinds that gently cleanse you. Exhale the negativity. Maintain this for about three minutes.

CORIANDER
(Coriandrum sativum)
PART USED: dried fruits, essential oil
PLANET: Mars
ELEMENT: Fire
MAGICAL INFLUENCES: Memory, Love, Healing
LORE:

Unlike the origins of many planet names, the etymology of coriander isn't filled with romance and intrigue. It stems from *koros*, a classical word meaning "bug."

Here in the Southwestern United States, the fresh leaves are often added to Mexican and Southeast Asian cooking. Many persons dislike their rather astringent, pungent taste and odor but the dried fruits are deliciously scented.

It was one of the first herbs I ever grew from seed.

MAGICAL USES:

In *The Art of Simpling*, an early treatise on herbalism, William Coles tells us to smell coriander to be ingenious and to have a good memory. The scent is also helpful in relieving headaches.

Crush a few of the small, round seeds between your fingers and sniff them while visualizing yourself in a loving, interpersonal relationship.

Or, inhale the odor of the crushed fruits and visualize it speeding up your body's healing processes.

COSTMARY
(Tanacetum balsamita)
PART USED: fresh and dried leaves
PLANET: Mercury

ELEMENT: Air
MAGICAL INFLUENCES: Conscious mind, Stilling
   emotions, Purification

I recently called a friend of mine in desperate search of
costmary. She generously gave me several large leaves
which she'd harvested from the plants in her garden.

Costmary is a unique herb with a unique scent. In
her monumental work, *A Modern Herbal*, M. Grieve
describes costmary's fragrance as being softly balsamic,
whereas to me this herb is warmly mint-like, not as
cool as peppermint but with the same basic scent. It is
quite agreeable.

I've never seen the dried herb for sale, but the
plants can be obtained through mail-order nurseries
(see Appendix II).

Sniff the leaves to awaken your conscious mind.
The fragrance, so refreshing and clean, clears away
mental fatigue, giving you a fresh start.

Additionally, smell costmary to calm raging emotions of all kinds—anger, fear, hatred, jealousy, obses-
sive love, pride and all those other wonderful feelings
that tell us we're alive.

Or, smell the scent of costmary leaves to purify
your inner self. Visualize it washing you clean.

CUMIN
(Cuminum cyminum)

PART USED: dried fruits
PLANET: Mars
ELEMENT: Fire
MAGICAL INFLUENCES: Protection
LORE:
   The fruits (often called seeds) are small, crescent-

shaped and have a spicy smell. They are much used in Mexican cooking because of their taste.

Cumin's aroma has long been thought to possess magical powers. In the 16th century, for example, William Coles wrote in his *Art of Simpling* that:

> "If one that hath eaten *Cumin* do but breathe on a painted face, the color will vanish away straight."

An odor thought to be strong enough to melt cosmetics was (and still is) a powerful force.

MAGICAL USES:
Crush some whole cumin and place in the top of a potpourri simmerer while visualizing your home as a safe, secure place, guarded against thieves and those who would harm you. As the water simmers and releases its fragrance in the air (which may take from ten to 20 minutes), the energies within the cumin will rise with the aroma and steam. Stay in the room. When you first smell it again, strongly visualize the home as a guarded, protected place. Repeat weekly or even daily as the need dictates.

Sniff the crushed seeds to internalize personal protection.

CYPRESS
(Cupressus sempervirens)
PART USED: essential oil
PLANET: Saturn
ELEMENT: Earth
MAGICAL INFLUENCES: Easing losses, Healing

The rather astringent scent of cypress oil is excellent

for smoothing transitions of all kinds, particularly the loss of friends and loved ones or the endings of relationships. Inhale the essential oil to find strength and comfort.

The cypress has long been planted in cemeteries throughout the Mediterranean region. It is an ancient symbol of comfort and solace, and its essential oil bestows this in time of need.

It is also protective to pets, since it "banishes" fleas from dogs, but don't anoint them with the undiluted essential oil. Place a few drops on the animal's bedding.

DAFFODIL
(*Narcissus* spp.)
PART USED: fresh flowers
PLANET: Venus
ELEMENT: Water
MAGICAL INFLUENCES: Love

These flowers in the narcissus family have faint, rather peculiar odors. Plant the bulbs in order to experience the joyous display of their flowers in the spring.

The aroma of fresh daffodil flowers instills spiritual love. Inhale the scent with proper visualizations.

DEERSTONGUE
(*Liatris odoratissimus; Frasera speciosa*)
PART USED: dried leaves
PLANET: Mars
ELEMENT: Fire
MAGICAL INFLUENCES: Psychic awareness

Deerstongue has a delicious, vanilla-like odor, thanks

to the coumarin contained with the plant—the same substance that gives woodruff and sweetgrass similar fragrances.

Crush the dried leaves between your fingers and inhale the odor to awaken your psychic awareness. This is especially effective late at night. Have your tarot cards, crystal sphere, rune stones or any other tools ready to use when you sit down with the deerstongue. Let psychic awareness blossom.

Some consider the scent to be sexually arousing to men.

DILL
(Anethum graveolens)

PART USED: fresh or dried fruits, leaves
PLANET: Mercury
ELEMENT: Air
MAGICAL INFLUENCES: Conscious mind, Purification

LORE:

No one who has ever smelled fresh dill will forget its scent. It is richer and more potent than that of the dried leaves or of pickles. Just smelling dill makes me hungry.

As far back as Culpeper's time (see Bibliography), the scent of dill was thought to "stayeth" hiccoughs.

MAGICAL USES:

The sharp odor (especially of fresh dill) sharpens the conscious mind. Smell it for a few seconds to clear your head. Then get on with the mental work at hand. This is ideal for balancing checkbooks.

If you enjoy the odor, inhale it during purification rituals while visualizing yourself being cleansed.

•

Taken internally, dill seed is considered to be an aphrodisiac. The aroma is not.

EUCALYPTUS
(Eucalyptus globulus)

PART USED: fresh leaves and seed pods, essential oil
PLANET: Mercury
ELEMENT: Air
MAGICAL INFLUENCES: Health, Purification, Healing

One of the great glories of living in southern California is the huge stands of eucalyptus trees all around us. Imported from Australia as windbreaks for orange groves, these fragrant, tall trees live on even after it was discovered that they topple over in a stiff breeze.

The scent of eucalyptus is crisp and well known from its widespread use in common cold preparations such as cough drops.

Inhale the fresh, camphor-like scent to maintain or regain health. Add a few drops to a potpourri simmerer (see Chapter 5) to purify (heal) a room or house of negative psychic energy, particularly when people have been engaged in verbal, emotional or physical combat.

Smell the crushed fresh leaves or fresh seed pods to induce health and to speed the healing process. A bunch of fresh leaves in a sickroom is also helpful.

FENNEL
(Foeniculum vulgare)

PART USED: fresh and dried seeds, essential oil
PLANET: Mercury

ELEMENT: Air
MAGICAL INFLUENCES: Longevity, Courage, Purification

LORE:

The fresh stalks were woven into chaplets with which Greek athletes were crowned. Fennel was also worn during public religious festivals in those times.

MAGICAL USES:

Masses of this vibrantly green plant grow in wastelands all over the country, especially here in southern California. In the summer, when the Sun bakes the drying seeds and stalks, the licorice-like fragrance rises on the hot air.

Inhaling the fragrance of fresh (or dried and crushed) fennel seeds is thought to increase the lifespan.

To produce courage, visualize and smell the essential oil or the herb itself. Vary your visualization to purify your inner self.

Warning: Bitter fennel essential oil has been determined to be hazardous. Use with caution and do not take internally.

FRANKINCENSE
(Boswellia carterii)
AKA: "Olibanum"

PART USED: essential oil
PLANET: Sun
ELEMENT: Air
MAGICAL EFFECTS: Spirituality, Meditation

Frankincense has 3,000 years of continuous magical and religious usage.

To produce a heightened awareness of the spiritual realms which lie hidden within the physical, or to deepen any religious experience, inhale the odor of this essential oil.

The aroma of frankincense also reduces stress and tension—not by revealing that the physical world is illusion (ask the tax man if it is) but by pointing out that our lives are bound up with more than one "reality." This knowledge is soothing in the face of adversity and hardship.

Inhaling the scent of frankincense essential oil calms the physical form and awakens higher consciousness. It is ideal for use prior to meditation.

Though "frankincense" oils are commonly sold in occult supply stores, don't anoint yourself with true, undiluted frankincense essential oil. It can irritate the skin.

FREESIA
(Freesia spp.)
PART USED: fresh flowers
PLANET: Venus
ELEMENT: Water
MAGICAL INFLUENCES: Love, Peace

In spring, these small flowers burst from the ground into riots of color. They produce a light, sweet fragrance. Ask for them at flower shops during spring or grow your own, since they must be used fresh and no essential oil is available.

Sniff freesias while visualizing yourself in a loving relationship. Let their energies mix with your own, transforming you into a person ready and willing to become involved in a satisfying relationship.

The power that rides on the scent transforms doubts about the possibility of love into positive, attracting energies.

When you're tense, the fragrance unknits the knots in your body and your mental state. Even the appearance of the flowers is cheering to the soul.

GALANGAL
(Alpina officinalis or *Galangal alpina)*
PART USED: dried root
PLANET: Mars
ELEMENT: Fire
MAGICAL INFLUENCES: Magical energy, Protection

Our name for this close relative of culinary ginger stems from the Arabic *Khalanjan.*

Galangal is usually sold in two forms: small, whole roots or slices of larger roots. Grind or break them apart before using.

Galangal possesses a stimulating scent akin to ginger. Inhale the fragrance prior to any type of magical working to increase your ability to draw personal energy from your body.

The scent is also useful to stave off the desire for sleep if you must keep working on a project. (Do remember, however, that nothing is a substitute for sleep!)

Additionally, the spicy odor is, with proper visualization, inhaled for personal protection.

The scent of galangal was once used to stimulate sexual desire but its effects, if any, seem to have been the product of suggestion rather than any direct physiological action.

GARDENIA
(Gardenia spp.)
PART USED: fresh flowers
PLANET: Moon
ELEMENT: Water
MAGICAL INFLUENCES: Peace, Love, Spirituality

The fragrance of fresh gardenia flowers is unforgettable. Sweet, powerful energies rise from the moon-drenched blooms.

Smell fresh gardenias to unwind after a busy day. Smell with visualization to find a love or to magnify the love you share with another. To spread loving energies throughout your home, place the fresh flowers in water in every room.

The white, round blooms of the gardenia are symbolically linked with the Moon. On the nights of the Full Moon, place cut gardenias in vases of water. Sit before them (in moonlight, if possible) and inhale the delicious fragrance to instill spirituality and to link with lunar energies.

Dried, the petals have a fragrance reminiscent of strawberry jam.

True gardenia absolute isn't currently available.

GARLIC
(Allium sativum)
PART USED: fresh cloves, fresh flowers
PLANET: Mars
ELEMENT: Fire
MAGICAL INFLUENCE: Protection, Purification, Health, Physical energy, Conscious mind

The powerful scent of fresh garlic is, as the old herbalists were apt to say, "too well knowne to need description." There are lovers and there are haters of this innocent plant, and they never seem to agree. However, garlic has a long and colorful history in magic and its permeating scent certainly has a place in magical aromatherapy.

If you enjoy the taste and especially the smell of garlic, use it as needed. If you detest "the stinking bulb," substitute some other aroma for the following uses.

To use, peel a fresh clove of garlic. If you have access to garlic plants, cut one flowerhead from the plant and place in water as usual. Garlic flowers are attractive and have a more subdued form of the characteristic scent.

Protection: Visualize the aroma wrapping around you, repelling negative energies.

Purification: Breathe in the stinging odor while visualizing it sweeping you clean of negative thoughts, of depression and of all forms of obsession.

Health: If you eat fresh garlic every day, as we've often been encouraged to do, sniff it (while visualizing its health-giving energies mingling with your body) before eating it.

Physical energy: When you're dragging around, smell the sharp, intense odor. Visualize sunshine or fiery rays of light sinking into your body through your nose. It'll really get you going.

Conscious mind: To stimulate thought processes and to encourage mental awareness, *lightly* inhale the scent.

Remember: Don't used dried or dehydrated garlic (or that adulterated substance known as "garlic salt"). Use the real thing.

GERANIUM

(Pelargonium graveolens)
AKA: "Rose Geranium"
PART USED: essential oil, fresh leaves
PLANET: Venus
ELEMENT: Water
MAGICAL INFLUENCES: Happiness, Protection

This essential oil isn't extracted from geraniums but from an entirely different genus of plants. The *Pelargoniums* are capable of imitating an amazing number of fragrances. Lemon, lime, nutmeg, peppermint, ginger, apple and apricot species are available. The essential oil labeled "Geranium" is usually made from the plant noted above—*Pelargonium graveolens*, rose geranium.

The fresh leaves or the essential oil can be used. Geranium is a rich, green, rose-like scent. Simply inhaling it calms the body and psyche, and refreshes it at the same time. This may be one of the reasons why it is used for protection.

When do we become ill? When our bodies' natural defenses have been depleted or subdued due to overwork, depression and a host of other causes. At such times we need to be "protected" against opportunistic viruses.

Similarly, we're most likely to be physically or "psychically" attacked when we're at our weakest. To give yourself a boost, put a few drops of geranium oil onto a cotton ball or bruise a fresh leaf and inhale the pleasing aroma. Let its energies wash over and through you, spreading peace and dissolving depression.

Visualize the fragrance healing your work- or world-weary soul. See it girding up your defenses against unwanted, outside, negative energy.

Simply getting in control of our lives is one of the most powerful defenses we can achieve, and geranium can help us to manifest this goal. We can't be sure of ourselves if we're depleted and feeling blue.

If you wish, put a few drops of the oil in a diffusor (see Chapter 5) and allow it to spread the scent throughout your home to guard it as well. Visualize the desired result, of course.

This is an easy plant to grow if you live in a warm climate, and it does well indoors as well. Buy a plant (see Appendix II), grow it and harvest a leaf or two as needed after the plant has reached a healthy size.

GINGER
(Zingiber officinale)

PART USED: fresh root, essential oil
PLANET: Mars
ELEMENT: Fire
MAGICAL INFLUENCES: Magical energy, Physical energy, Sex, Love, Money, Courage

The scent of fresh ginger (or the essential oil) may surprise those who have only encountered the spice in its dried, powdered form. Many grocery stores offer fresh ginger in the produce section. Culinary ginger is even grown on a commercial scale in the United States—on the Big Island of Hawaii.

The essential oil has a somewhat more bitter scent than the fresh root, but the spiciness is definitely there.

Inhale the biting fragrance before magical rituals

of all kinds, visualizing it stimulating the physical body, exciting muscular contraction and thereby producing bioelectrical energy. This same effect of ginger can be used to provide a temporary storehouse of extra energy when needed. (However, nothing—including drugs or essential oils—can replace natural sleep.)

In his classic text, *The Practice of Aromatherapy*, Jean Valnet says that the women of Senegal wear (or wore) belts of ginger roots to sexually arouse their husbands. This is no surprise, for the spicy, zingy scent of ginger has long been used to create sexual desire. Its effect may be more psychological than physiological but if it helps, it helps. Remember: inhale with appropriate visualization.

For centuries, ginger has been used in love rituals throughout Asia and the South Pacific. Originally introduced as an exotic condiment in Europe, ginger was soon used for both medicinal as well as amatory purposes. This ancient heritage is recognized in the extensive use of ginger in men's colognes, though at the moment sweeter, less spicy formulas are being created for the scent-conscious man.

Ginger was once worth more than its weight in gold. Its pungent scent is appropriate for bringing money into your life. Sniff and visualize.

Ginger also promotes courage, confidence, aggression (which is necessary to self-survival), purification and success on all levels. Because of its active, vibrant nature, it's best not to sniff this scent directly prior to going to bed (unless you're not planning on immediately going to sleep . . .).

GINGER, WHITE
(Hedychium coronarium)

PART USED: fresh flowers
PLANET: Venus
ELEMENT: Water
MAGICAL INFLUENCES: Purification, Love, Peace
LORE:

Early visitors to Hawaii will remember the deliciously sweet scent of white ginger flowers. A native of India, this was the most popular lei flower in Hawaii until the end of World War II. The fields on Oahu where this plant was cultivated were covered with houses in the post-war building boom. The plumeria, carnation and tuberose soon replaced it. Today, white ginger leis are only found in a few lei stands, carefully refrigerated and quite expensive. But the plant grows wild on lower elevations and flourishes around the steam vents near Volcano House on the Big island of Hawaii.

MAGICAL USES:

This plant, a true member of the ginger family, somewhat resembles bamboo or banana until it unfurls butterfly shaped, exotically scented flowers. The roots have the characteristic gingerish scent, but the flowers betray none of this spiciness. This is a good example of the way in which specific parts of a plant contain different essential oils and, thus, varying scents.

Like many others, I first discovered this flower in Hawaii and was fortunate enough to find starter plants at a local nursery. I gave them to my mother and now her plants produce hundreds of exquisite blooms every year.

White ginger, as with most heavenly scented flowers, stimulates love and creates peace. It is a soothing aroma. The delicate scent can also be used for internal purification.

The plants can be difficult to find and the flowers are never sold, save in Hawaii, where white ginger leis can occasionally be found. If someone you know is going there, ask them to bring you back a string of these exquisite flowers and experiment. (A mail-order source for starter plants is included in Appendix II.)

Though perfumes bearing this name can be found, no true white ginger essential oil is currently available.

HONEYSUCKLE
(Lonicera caprifolium)

PART USED: fresh flowers, absolute
PLANET: Jupiter
ELEMENT: Earth
MAGICAL INFLUENCES: Weight loss, Psychic awareness, Prosperity

The luxuriant sweetness of honeysuckle can, surprisingly enough, be used to encourage weight loss.

Collect one or two flowering strands of honeysuckle with thanks. Place them in a jar of water. Stand or sit before the flowers (within nose reach) and visualize the way you'll look after losing the weight. Intensify the visualization and inhale the odor. Whenever you feel the urge to ruin your diet or to ignore your exercise routine (if any), once again go to the flowers and drink in their scent with visualization.

Honeysuckle can also be inhaled to strengthen psychic awareness. Sit quietly and allow its scent to lull your conscious mind into breaking its grip on your psychic mind.

Long used for increasing money in folk magic, the sweet aroma can be inhaled with visualization to manifest the sweet scent of money.

HOPS
(Humulus lupulus)
PART USED: fresh and dried flowers
PLANET: Mars
ELEMENT: Air
MAGICAL INFLUENCES: Sleep, Healing

Today, many people only encounter hops in bottles of beer, but this strangely named and strangely shaped plant was once the most-prescribed tranquilizer. Sniffing the scent of the fresh or dried flowers brings on natural sleep. Small pillows can be made of the dried flowers.

Or, just before bedtime, inhale the scent and visualize it strengthening and maintaining your health. Let the hop energy do its work as you sleep.

This ritual is fine at all times of day, but be warned that its scent is calming and relaxing.

HYACINTH
(Hyacinthus orientalis)
PART USED: fresh flowers
PLANET: Venus
ELEMENT: Water
MAGICAL INFLUENCES: Overcoming grief, Love, Peaceful sleep

This plant is a popular spring bloomer. The delicious

fragrance of the flowers was once commonly inhaled to halt consuming grief. If this is a problem, visualize yourself as a poised, confident person and sniff the flowers. Repeat this two or three times a day until the situation has been corrected.

As with all flowers ruled by Venus, the fragrance of hyacinth can be used in rituals designed to bring love into your life.

One legendary property of this scent: it halts nightmares. Place a blooming plant beside the bed so that the room fills with its fragrance at night. Drop off to sleep smelling the scent and visualizing a good night's sleep. No bizarre dreams should disturb your rest.

HYSSOP
(Hyssopus officinalis)

PART USED: fresh leaves, essential oil
PLANET: Jupiter
ELEMENT: Fire
MAGICAL INFLUENCES: Purification, Conscious mind

Hyssop has long been used in ritual. Temples in ancient Greece were swept with bunches of this herb. Hyssop was deemed to be sacred to the goddesses and gods.

Inhale the sharp, greenly-scented essential oil for purification. Or, sniff sprigs of the fresh herb. Place hyssop in a vase of water and leave in the home to purify it as well.

Because of its associations with religion, the scent of fresh hyssop can be sniffed to heighten spirituality prior to religious rituals of all kinds.

Sniff fresh hyssop to clear your head and to

strengthen mental processes.

Warning: Hyssop essential oil is a highly potent form of this herb. It is toxic in large doses. According to the literature, it should not be used by women during pregnancy, or by epileptics. Valnet (see Bibliography) quotes expert sources as saying that this may be the only essential oil capable of producing true epileptic attack. For safety, substitute the fresh herb.

IRIS
(Iris florentina)
AKA: "Orris" (the rootstock)
PART USED: the dried, prepared root
PLANET: Venus
ELEMENT: Water
MAGICAL INFLUENCES: Love, Psychic awareness

This plant was named after the Greek goddess of the Rainbow, Iris.

Dried and cured "orris" root possesses a unique, violet-like fragrance which has long been associated with love. In American folk magic, the ground root is sprinkled onto bedsheets and onto the body to induce amorous feelings.

Inhale the sweet fragrance of orris root during love rituals of all kinds.

Additionally, sniff this aroma (with visualization, as always) to facilitate a connection between your psychic and conscious minds.

JASMINE
(Jasminum grandiflorum)
(Jasminum officinale)
(Jasminum sambac)

PART USED: Fresh flowers, absolute
PLANET: Moon
ELEMENT: Water
MAGICAL INFLUENCES: Love, Peace, Spirituality, Sex, Sleep, Psychic dreams

Jasmine (together with rose and neroli) has the honor of being one of the highest-priced plant scents. One or two milliliters of true jasmine absolute currently sells for $40.00 and up.

Jasmine is an exquisitely expensive, exquisitely delightful aromatic.

Perhaps 99 per cent of all "oil of jasmine" sold today is synthetic. This can easily be determined by the sickly sweet, chemical odor of such products as well as the cheap price. Cost and your nose will determine if the product is true jasmine.

An alternative to these costly substances are fresh jasmine flowers, but many of the plants sold as jasmine (such as night-blooming jasmine) aren't even in the same family. Only those plants listed above should be used for magical aromatherapy purposes. If all else fails, buy a small sample of true jasmine absolute and sparingly use it.

Jasmine has often been called the king of flowers ("as rose is the queen"). This is perhaps because the absolute is surprisingly dark-hued. Some experts detect animal-like undertones in it, and in *The Art of Aromatherapy*, Robert Tisserand classifies jasmine as a yang (masculine) plant.

In China, however, the fragrant flowers are symbolic of women. Traditional aromatherapists utilize jasmine to alleviate women's reproductive problems and to facilitate childbirth. Moreover, the beautiful blossoms and the delicious scent seem more related to feminine energy in general.

Therefore, in direct opposition to aromatherapy tradition, I've classified jasmine as a feminine (yin) plant, ruled by the Moon and possessed of the qualities of the element of Water.

Because of the intensity of the odor, its scarcity and high cost, one drop of jasmine absolute on a cotton ball is sufficient for the uses listed below.

Jasmine's powerful scent directly affects our emotional centers, making it an excellent choice for use in love rituals. Inhale the aroma with proper visualizations to enhance an ongoing relationship or to find a new one.

This beautiful fragrance lifts our spirits, dispels depression, quiets nerves and stifles worries about tomorrow. You needn't visualize to reap these changes—simply breathe.

Jasmine's calming, soothing fragrance is also of tremendous help in relaxing our physical bodies.

This scent can lull us into states of heightened spiritual awareness with the proper visualization. Be aware of the divine energy which is manifested within the odor. Breathe it in and connect with the energy behind all in existence.

One of the most celebrated uses of jasmine absolute is in inducing sexual desire. With proper visualization, the aroma of jasmine creates the mental, emotional and physical responses necessary for sexual arousal.

Jasmine is also used to treat emotional sexual dysfunction (in women, the inability to enjoy sexual contact or to achieve orgasm; in men, the same two conditions as well as difficulty in achieving or maintaining erection and lack of ejaculation). Sniff and visualize.

To encourage sleep, sniff the absolute oil. This may also produce psychic dreams.

The scent and potential uses of jasmine absolute far outweigh the high cost of the substance.

JUNIPER
(Juniperus communis)

PART USED: essential oil, dried fruit
PLANET: Sun
ELEMENT: Fire
MAGICAL EFFECTS: Protection, Purification, Healing
LORE:

Juniper was burned to goddesses and gods in ancient Sumer and Babylon, and was widely used in Egyptian incense formulas. It was sacred to Inanna and her later counterpart Ishtar. Many centuries later in Europe, branches of juniper were smouldered and carried around fields and farms to release protective energies and to guard livestock and crops.

It is a common ritual incense ingredient in Tibet and was much used by various American Indian groups.

MAGICAL USES:

Juniper essential oil is currently used in traditional aromatherapy to detoxify the body, as a parasiticide (parasite destroyer) and antiseptic. This seems in keeping with the "magical" use of purifying homes and fields mentioned above, for protective rituals are designed to ward off negativity as well as to purge such energies from a person or place.

Inhale juniper essential oil while visualizing its energies guarding you from negativity and danger.

Or, for an internal purification, smell juniper and visualize.

You can also make juniper a part of health-maintaining rituals. Regularly smell the scent while seeing yourself eating correctly, exercising and thinking positively.

LAVENDER
(Lavendula officinalis)

PART USED: fresh flowers, dried flowers, essential oil

PLANET: Mercury

ELEMENT: Air

MAGICAL INFLUENCES: Health, Love, Celibacy, Peace, Conscious mind

LORE:

Well known to the classical Greeks and Romans, lavender was used to perfume bath water and was burned as incense to the deities.

In North Africa, women used this plant to guard against maltreatment from their husbands.

The scent is said to calm untamed lions and tigers.

MAGICAL USES:

Just before you step into the water, add nine drops of lavender essential oil to your bath while visualizing good health. Have a lavender bath once daily for a week as a health-maintaining ritual.

Lavender has long been associated with spiritual love. Because it is ruled by Mercury, the planet associated with the conscious mind, lavender's effectiveness in promoting love seems to lie in its ability to change the way we think about love. In other words, performing love-drawing rituals with lavender stimulates the emotional centers and, thereby, reprograms our conscious minds. Smelling lavender with visualization causes us to send signals to others of our need.

The scent can also be used to maintain celibacy with the proper visualization. Though the complete lack of sexual thoughts or sexual activity (even if performed alone) is contrary to the human experience, there are times when it may be necessary. Lavender can be used to help create this precarious state.

Lavender induces peace and dispels depression. The fragrance has been used for this purpose from very early times. Gerard states that "the distilled water of Lavendar smelt unto, or the temples and forehead bathed therewith, is refreshing to them . . . that used to swoune much." It relieves headache as well.

Lavender calms stormy or uncontrolled emotional states by bringing our feelings under conscious control. Too often when we're in such states we kill off all thoughts save for those that prolong our misery. Lavender corrects this imbalance, tempering our emotions with a healthy shot of rationality. The fragrance is also used to generally strengthen the conscious mind. (I should have used it when I was trying to compute the tab for an essential oil order I wrote up yesterday afternoon.)

Sprinkled on the pillow, it encourages sleep.

LEMON
(Citrus limonum)

PART USED: essential oil, fresh zest
PLANET: Moon
ELEMENT: Water
MAGICAL INFLUENCES: Health, Healing, Physical
    energy, Purification

The essential oil, cold pressed from the outer rind of lemons, has the crisp, clean scent of the fruit itself.

If you can't obtain the essential oil, simply grate off the colored "skin" of one lemon, wrap in a thin cotton cloth, squeeze and inhale for the following uses. (What to do with the nude lemon? Squeeze it, dilute its juice with water and drink, preferably without sugar, for its general tonic action on the physical body. Evidence suggests that lemon juice, taken internally, stimulates white corpuscles to fight off infections. It is also mildly stimulating.)

Inhale the refreshing scent to maintain health and as an adjunct to conventional medical treatment. Visualize its energies strengthening your body as well as the two minds that control it. In the case of illness, see the fragrance fighting off the infection. For wounds, visualize the aroma encouraging cell growth and the resultant healing.

The lively scent also activates the body, dispelling sluggishness. Inhaling fresh lemon zest or the essential oil first thing in the morning is the aromatic substitute for a cup of coffee. Visualize its fragrance revitalizing and stimulating the central nervous system.

Additionally, inhale the aroma for purification.

Place a few drops into a diffusor or potpourri simmerer and feel the energies of your home vibrate and hum with purity.

Adding undiluted lemon essential oil to the bath or rubbing it into the skin will cause irritation and is best avoided.

LEMON BALM
(Melissa officinalis)
AKA: "Melissa"

PART USED: fresh leaves, essential oil
PLANET: Jupiter
ELEMENT: Air
MAGICAL INFLUENCES: Peace, Money, Purification
LORE:

For centuries, wooden furniture was rubbed with fresh lemon balm leaves not only to produce a shine but also to drive out "evil spirits."

The fresh leaves have been rubbed onto hives to attract bees since at least Roman times.

According to ancient instructions (as quoted in Kamm), the whole plant, including the root, stems, leaves and flowers, was dried, sewn into a piece of linen with silk thread and worn under the clothing. This made its bearer "beloved and agreeable to those one met," fulfilled every desire and ensured perpetual happiness. A tall order, considering the size of a mature plant.

MAGICAL USES:

The dried leaves are virtually worthless for magical aromatherapy even though they retain a slight scent. The fresh leaves (or essential oil) are necessary for the following uses.

Both the fresh and essential oil forms of lemon balm possess a crisp, lemony odor remarkably similar to that of the true lemon. This fragrance is sedative by nature. It releases muscular tension and lulls our racing minds. Because of this action it often produces an uplifting feeling which mellows into a quiet peace. The scent of lemon balm is also inhaled with visualization to relieve depression and to calm raging emotions.

As far back as Culpeper's time (see Bibliography) it was known for its uplifting properties. It "driveth away all troublesome cares and thoughts out of the mind," the famous herbalist wrote.

Those of us experiencing money problems should be aware that we've created this situation. Inhale lemon balm's delightful fragrance while visualizing yourself allowing money into your life. This works by removing blockages we've set up within ourselves against receiving money. We may not be consciously aware of these blockages but they're there.

This scent is so crisp and clean that it can be inhaled as part of a daily or weekly personal purification ritual.

Lemon balm essential oil (also known as Melissa) is expensive, and is difficult to find in a pure, unadulterated form.

Warning: Lemon balm essential oil may cause allergic reactions.

LEMONGRASS
(Cymbopogon citratus)
PART USED: essential oil, fresh or dried leaves
PLANET: Mercury
ELEMENT: Air

MAGICAL INFLUENCES: Psychic awareness, Purification

Lemongrass is popularly used in Asian, Mexican and
South American cooking. It has an intense lemon
odor.

The scent has been found to stimulate psychic
awareness through inhalation and visualization. Break
apart the dried herb (or rub the fresh herb with your
fingers) to release the fragrance. Inhale and awaken
your psychic mind.

Like all lemon-scented plants and essential oils,
lemongrass essential oil can be used for personal
purification rituals. But don't add it to the bath. It is
irritating to the skin.

LEMON VERBENA
(Lippia citriodora)
AKA: "Verbena"
PART USED: fresh leaves, essential oil
PLANET: Mercury
ELEMENT: Air
MAGICAL INFLUENCES: Love, Purification

All these "lemon" plants and their essential oils are
often confused. Lemon verbena is even more likely to
be misnamed, as some believe the plant (especially by
the name verbena) to be identical with Vervain (*Verbena officinalis*), an entirely different plant. True lemon
verbena essential oil is expensive and, not surprisingly, has the familiar scent.

The fresh leaves, when you can obtain them (see
why you should grow herbs?), are far less costly. This
herb has been used to excite spiritual love since it was

brought from its native Chile to Europe about 200 years ago. Crush the fresh leaves or inhale the essential oil and visualize.

It is also a wonderful purifier, inhaled or added to a diffusor. But don't add the essential oil to your bathwater.

LILAC
(Syringa vulgaris)
PART USED: fresh flowers
PLANET: Venus
ELEMENT: Earth
MAGICAL INFLUENCES: Love, Purification

The scent of fresh lilac flowers was once thought to drive away ghosts.

Like many flowers, lilacs can be utilized in love-expansion rituals. The sweet fragrance of these seasonal blooms brims with loving energies.

Or, inhale the aroma rising from the light purple flowers for internal purification. To cleanse a home, place jars of the fresh flowers in several rooms.

Lilacs are scarce around these parts, since most species must freeze in order to produce blooms. Still, I manage to smell the flowers once or twice yearly.

No true lilac essential oil is currently available.

LILY
(Lilium spp.)
PART USED: fresh flowers
PLANET: Moon
ELEMENT: Water
MAGICAL INFLUENCES: Peace, Easing pain of broken relationships

LORE:

I've found much lore regarding the noble lily, once dedicated to the Goddess throughout Europe (in Crete, to Britomartis; Greece, to Hera; Rome, to Juno). It was later sanitized and "converted" to symbolize the Virgin Mary.

The Fragrant Garden by Wilder (see Bibliography) records many curious ideas concerning lilies. The scent itself, though sweet, was thought to be injurious to the health if inhaled for long periods of time. Even death was thought to have resulted when persons slept in a room filled with fresh lilies.

To foretell the sex of a child, persons once approached a pregnant woman with a lily in one hand and a rose in the other. If she chose the lily, she would have a son. If the rose, a daughter.

The lily is the flower of choice for symbolizing the ancient Pagan Spring festival in its current Christianized form of Easter.

MAGICAL USES:

The lily's long association with feminine spirituality seems to make it ideal for those women unshackling themselves from the effects of patriarchal society. Not being a woman, I don't know what effects the scent of this flower may manifest. A suggestion: sniff, attune with ancient feminine spirituality (the Goddess). See yourself as an active, alive woman, in control of your life. Repeat whenever you feel patriarchy crushing down upon you.

The scent of lilies is also soothing and imbues its admirer with peaceful feelings.

A specific use of the sweet fragrance is to quench

the pain of a broken, once loving relationship. Frequently inhale the aroma while visualizing yourself as a happy, well-adjusted individual who can get along just fine without her or him. Once you've achieved this state, begin a love ritual utilizing one of the many essential oils or plants useful for this purpose.

LILY OF THE VALLEY
(Convallaria magalis)
PART USED: fresh flowers
PLANET: Mercury
ELEMENT: Air
MAGICAL INFLUENCES: Peace, Conscious mind, Memory

Apollo was credited with finding this plant and presenting it to Aesculapius.

The well-known and dangerous effects of lily of the valley apply to its internal use, but not to its fragrance. Once again, don't eat, drink, add to your bath water or rub onto your skin any substance that you're not specifically directed to use in these ways. Just a reminder!

This tiny plant produces sprays of white, bell-shaped flowers that emit what Culpeper calls a "pleasant, grateful scent." The aroma instills peace and strengthens the conscious mind. With visualization, the scent will heighten your ability to recall old information and strengthen your powers of memory.

The flowers have to be harvested to be used for these purposes. The last time I smelled lily of the valley I got down on all fours, stuck my left ear onto the Earth and sniffed away. Not exactly a position that induces calm.

Though the cut flowers are occasionally available in florist establishments in springtime, no true lily of the valley essential oil is available.

LIME
(Citrus aurantifolia)

PART USED: essential oil, fresh zest

PLANET: Sun

ELEMENT: Fire

MAGICAL INFLUENCES: Purification, Physical energy, Protection

The true essential oil captures the pungent citrus scent of the fruit. To use the zest, grate off the colored portion of a ripe lime, enclose in a thin cloth and squeeze just before inhaling.

The scent of lime is curiously similar to and yet so different from that of lemon. It is full-bodied, sharper and possesses a curious tweak that makes it instantly recognizable to anyone who's ever smelled the fresh fruit or peelings.

Like all citrusy scents, it is effective in personal purification. The powerful aroma (ruled by the Sun) also energizes and revitalizes the body.

It can be used, with the appropriate visualizations, for personal protection.

MACE
(Myristica fragrans)

PART USED: Mace is the red membrane covering the kernels of the fruits of the nutmeg tree

PLANET: Mercury

ELEMENT: Air

MAGICAL INFLUENCES: Psychic awareness

Mace emits a powerful, spicy odor and is well known from its use in cooking.

To enhance psychic awareness, sit comfortably and inhale this aroma, visualizing it penetrating your conscious mind, relaxing its hold and traveling to your deep consciousness. Psychic awareness will blossom.

MAGNOLIA
(Magnolia spp.)
PART USED: fresh flowers
PLANET: Venus
ELEMENT: Water
MAGICAL INFLUENCES: Love

Magnolia has long been a symbol of feminine beauty in China. On my last trip to Louisiana, the blossoming trees lining the streets of Baton Rouge and New Orleans filled the air with a rich, heady fragrance.

Inhale the aroma of the fresh flowers to increase your ability to give and to receive love.

No true magnolia essential oil is available.

MARJORAM
(Origanum marjorana)
PART USED: fresh leaves and flowers, essential oil
PLANET: Mercury
ELEMENT: Air
MAGICAL INFLUENCES: Peace, Celibacy, Sleep
LORE:

Since Roman times, the scent of marjoram has been thought to convey longevity. The goddess Venus was said to have granted the plant its fragrance. A strange belief states that anyone foolish enough to smell marjoram would have her or his nose pulled off by the plant—an observation of its peppery scent.

MAGICAL USES:

This is a sedative aroma, useful in allaying anxiety and all agitated emotional states such as grief, love-obsession and our reactions to the passing of friends and loved ones. It is even useful in halting the desire for sexual contact.

It inclines to restful sleep. Over-inhalation of the scent can put you out like a light.

On a more spiritual level, smelling marjoram for a few seconds before any type of rite facilitates ritual consciousness (the unification of the psychic and conscious minds necessary for successful ritual). Inhaling the essential oil or the fresh herb for too long may mean you'll sleep through the ritual. Less is best.

Warning: Patricia Davis in *Aromatherapy: An A-Z*, warns that marjoram essential oil shouldn't be used by pregnant mothers to avoid possible injury to both parties.

MEADOWSWEET
(Spiraea filipendula)
PART USED: fresh leaves, dried leaves
PLANET: Jupiter
ELEMENT: Air
MAGICAL INFLUENCES: Peace, Love

Gerard states that the fragrance of meadowsweet "makes the heart merrie," won't cause headache or dull the appetite.

Long associated with love in European folk magic, the scent of meadowsweet can indeed be used to expand our ability to give and receive love. Inhale the aroma with visualization.

MELON
(various)
PART USED: fresh fruit
PLANET: Moon
ELEMENT: Water
MAGICAL INFLUENCES: Healing, Health

The scent of melons (especially cantaloupe, honeydew and other popular varieties) strengthens the body and hones its ability to heal itself or to maintain good health.

To accomplish these purposes, breathe in the fruity fragrance with visualization. See the delicious aroma building up your body, strengthening it, increasing its capacity to guard itself against opportunistic infections. Then eat the fruit to fully partake of its energies.

MIMOSA
(Acacia dealbata)
PART USED: fresh flowers
PLANET: Saturn
ELEMENT: Earth
MAGICAL INFLUENCES: Psychic dreams, Love

These round, yellow flowers emit a sweet scent which can produce psychic dreams. Inhale the odor as you go to sleep, visualizing it unlocking the door to your psychic mind. Then, in your dreams, receive glimpses of possible future events from your deep consciousness through the language of symbols.

Like most flowers, the scent can also be used with visualization to bring love.

MUGWORT
(Artemesia vulgaris)

PART USED: fresh leaves
PLANET: Venus
ELEMENT: Earth
MAGICAL INFLUENCES: Psychic awareness, Psychic dreams, Astral projection

This beautiful herb has long been associated with the shadowy world of the seer as well as with the Moon. Its scent stills the conscious mind and awakens the deep consciousness.

To promote psychic awareness, inhale the odor of the fresh, crushed leaves with visualization. For psychic dreams, inhale directly prior to falling asleep.

To utilize its legendary ability to effect astral projection (the separation of the consciousness from the body, allowing it to travel at will unbounded by distance or time), sniff before making the attempt while visualizing perfect control over this ability.

Warning: The essential oil is considered to be hazardous and is not recommended for use!

MYRRH
(Comniphora myrrha)

PART USED: essential oil, the oleo-gum-resin
PLANET: Saturn
ELEMENT: Water
MAGICAL INFLUENCES: Spirituality, Meditation, Healing

Myrrh possesses a richly bitter scent. This exotic substance has been used in magic and religion for at least 4,000 years.

Inhale the fragrance of the essential oil or the crushed resin (more properly, oleo-gum-resin) to awaken your awareness of the spiritual reality behind our everyday existence. This is an excellent tool to use prior to or during religious rituals. The resultant expanded awareness also calms fears and halts questions concerning the future.

Similarly, sniff myrrh prior to meditation to achieve a fitting mood. Or, inhale the richly bitter scent with visualization to speed healing of the physical body.

The essential oil is best for magical aromatherapy, for it releases a stronger aroma than the dried oleo-gum-resin.

NARCISSUS
(Narcissus spp.)

PART USED: fresh flowers
PLANET: Venus
ELEMENT: Water
MAGICAL INFLUENCES: Love
LORE AND LEGEND:

In China, for centuries, narcissi bulbs have been placed in bowls with rocks and water. They are "forced" into flowering by the Chinese New Year to acquire good fortune. The practice still continues throughout that huge country.

It may be that this plant wasn't named after the youth who fell in love with his reflection in a pool of water and drowned. Pliny states that the name was derived from the word *narkao*, to benumb, due to the plant's dramatic effects on the nervous system when taken internally. Never eat any part of this plant.

MAGICAL USES:

These beautiful flowers (the daffodil is also a Narcissus) emit sweet, lovely fragrances long used to manifest new relationships or to enrich the love already shared with another. The purple varieties seem to be best for this use.

In the Middle East, the scent is thought to be aphrodisiac.

NASTURTIUM
(*Nasturtium* spp.)

PART USED: fresh flowers
PLANET: Mars
ELEMENT: Fire
MAGICAL INFLUENCES: Physical energy, Protection

The name is derived from the Latin words *narsus* (nose) and *tortus* (twisted), or nose-twister. Pliny states that the smell of burning nasturtium drives away snakes.

I actually ate this flower before ever enjoying its bitter, peppery odor, and it tastes just as hot on the tongue. The powerful odor of nasturtiums lends us energy in times of physical demands. Smell the fresh flowers first thing on waking up. Even if you're too sleepy to visualize, you'll receive a great start on your day. The scent fully arouses your conscious mind and energizes the physical body.

Like black pepper, the scent can also be used with visualization to guard yourself or your home from physical attack and negative energy. Visualize its scent hovering around you (or your home) like an invisible shield.

NEROLI
(Citrus aurantium)
AKA: "Orange Blossom" "Orange Flower"
PART USED: essential oil
PLANET: Sun
ELEMENT: Fire
MAGICAL INFLUENCES: Purification, Joy, Sex

Neroli essential oil is distilled from the flowers of the bitter orange tree. It is incredibly expensive but well worth the cost, for its heady, rich scent is useful in achieving the following magical changes:

Self-purification. Inhale while visualizing the scent burning away negative thought-patterns, harmful habits and other misuses of your bioelectrical energy and mind.

Joy. Sniff the luxurious scent to lift your spirits and to at least temporarily settle emotional upsets. This is, in a sense, a form of self-purification. It may even create a feeling of euphoria.

Sexual relations. Inhale while visualizing your physical, emotional, spiritual, mental and psychic connection with the person in question. While not considered to be truly aphrodisiac in its effects, neroli essential oil calms the conscious mind, allays worries over sexual "performance" and smooths the path to mutually satisfying sexual relations.

In her excellent book *Aromatherapy: An A-Z*, Patricia Davis says that this effect of the scent of orange flowers explains why they've long been popular in bridal wreaths.

Neroli essential oil, while costly, has such a delicious odor that it's worth putting away money earmarked for its purchase.

NIAOULI
(Melaleuca viridiflora)
AKA: "Gomenol"

PART USED: essential oil
PLANET: Mercury
ELEMENT: Air
MAGICAL INFLUENCES: Protection, Healing

Not to be confused with neroli (see last entry), niaouli is a far different essential oil with an unusual scent. It resembles eucalyptus but has a rich, almost pine-like note. The aroma is fantastically refreshing and invigorating.

Niaouli essential oil is useful in overcoming "psychic attack," whether real or (as is usually the case) imagined. I define psychic attack as the conscious, willfull direction of negatively-charged energy toward a specific person with the intention of causing harm.

To combat psychic attack, perform the following rite upon waking, several times during the day and just before going to sleep.

Sit in a quiet place. Still your mind. Sprinkle a few drops of niaouli oil onto a cotton ball. Inhale the strong, fresh aroma. As you inhale, visualize its energies mixing with yours, forming an impenetrable barrier against all negative energies which may be directed toward you.

Continue to breathe in the fragrance until you feel you've done enough. When you're finished, place the cotton ball in a small plastic bag and carry it with you wherever you go. Whenever you feel the need throughout the day, use the same cotton ball for later repetitions of this simple but powerful ritual.

The scent of niaouli essential oil is not only refreshing and protective, but also stimulates our bodies to heal themselves. Inhale the aroma and visualize.

Inexpensively priced, niaouli oil is one of my favorites.

NUTMEG
(Myristica fragrans)

PART USED: dried kernel (nut) of the fruit, essential oil
PLANET: Jupiter
ELEMENT: Fire
MAGICAL INFLUENCES: Physical energy, Magical energy, Psychic awareness, Money

The state of Connecticut was once famous for nutmegs. Enterprising business persons whittled wood into the shape of this once costly spice and placed these "woodnuts" among shipments of the real thing to improve their profits while cheating their buyers.

Anyone who has ever had a sip of real eggnog knows the powerful spiciness of nutmegs The scent, so warming and stimulating to the physical body, is inhaled prior to any form of magic which requires a tremendous release of bioelectrical energy. Visualize its scent (and, hence its energy) mingling with and arousing your own in preparation for the coming magical act.

The fragrance of nutmeg is suited to bringing money into your life. Smell and visualize.

In herbal folk magic, nutmeg has long been utilized to tap into our psychic minds, and the scent can also be called upon for this purpose.

Warning: Nutmeg essential oil is toxic in large quantities. Do not inhale for long periods of time, and do not add to bathwater.

OAKMOSS
(Evernia prusnatri)
PART USED: the whole, dried plant
PLANET: Jupiter
ELEMENT: Earth
MAGICAL INFLUENCES: Money

The sweet, earthy scent of this lichen (it isn't a moss) has long been used in cosmetic perfumery. In magic oakmoss is called upon to increase cash flow and to expand personal prosperity.

To accomplish this, crush a bit of the greyish-yellowish herb between your fingers and inhale with visualization. Its earthy, spicy scent seems drenched with money energy.

An absolute of oakmoss is available.

ONION
(Allium cepa)
PART USED: fresh bulb
PLANET: Mars
ELEMENT: Fire
MAGICAL INFLUENCES: Courage, Protection

Some may find it strange to see this vegetable listed here, but its scent is so sharp that it must be included.

To bolster your courage, slice off the end of a fresh onion. Smell its stinging, powerful fragrance. Breathe it in (and wipe your eyes, if necessary), feeling it dissolving doubts about your abilities, firming up your resolution and giving you the courage to do what you must do.

The fragrance can also be used to protect your home. With a sharp knife, quarter fresh onions until you have one piece for every room of your home. Place one quarter in each room on a paper plate, visualizing the overpowering odor setting up a strong barrier against negativity.

Open the windows and doors (if the weather allows) and maintain your visualization for at least a few minutes.

Gather the onions and place them outside. The scent may lead your neighbors to think you're cooking up a storm. In a sense you are, by calling upon the forceful, projective energies of onions to safeguard your home.

Some consider the scent of fresh onion to be an aphrodisiac. This is an acquired, ah, taste.

ORANGE
(Citrus sinensis)

PART USED: fresh zest, essential oil
PLANET: Sun
ELEMENT: Fire
MAGICAL INFLUENCES: Purification, Joy, Physical energy, Magical energy

The colored portion of the peel or the essential oil releases the familiar, sweet, citrusy odor. Like neroli, this fragrance is ideal for self-purification, for transforming depression into peace or even joy, and for producing an increase in available bioelectrical energy when needed for both mundane and magical workings.

In larger amounts the scent may create the desire for sleep.

PALMAROSA
(Cymbopogon martini)

PART USED: essential oil
PLANET: Venus
ELEMENT: Water
MAGICAL INFLUENCES: Love, Healing

Palmarosa essential oil is steam distilled from a plant closely related to lemongrass. The essential oil has a citrus-rose scent which is refreshing and somewhat compelling.

Inhale palmarosa essential oil during love-attracting rituals with proper visualization. While not so strong as rose, jasmine and other aromas, it does its part in achieving your needed change. One point in its favor is its vastly lower price.

Palmarosa also speeds healing when used with visualization and, of course, proper treatment. Smell it at least once a day while visualizing your body in a healthy, healed, whole state.

Some don't like the scent of palmarosa. Its aroma is so unusual that it smells like a mixture. It is exotic and yet quite inexpensive.

PARSLEY
(Petroselinum sativum)

PART USED: fresh herb
PLANET: Mercury
ELEMENT: Air
MAGICAL INLUENCES: Protection

Those who are familiar with this herb only in its dried

form may be surprised by the aroma of the fresh plant. Among the unique qualities of this culinary herb is its ability to overcome strong scents such as garlic. Rubbing your hands with fresh parsley after handling garlic cloves will cleanse them of the smell.

Sniff fresh, bruised parsley with visualization to protect your home and yourself. Place bunches of the fresh leaves (available in markets everywhere) in glasses of water to spread its protective energies.

PATCHOULY
(Pogostemon patchouli)

PART USED: dried leaves, essential oil
PLANET: Saturn
ELEMENT: Earth
MAGICAL INFLUENCES: Sex, Physical energy, Money

Pity the poor, downtrodden patchouly. This aroma took a real dip in popularity after the psychedelic '60s, when adulterated patchouly was used to mask the odor of marijuana smoke. To this day, many people dislike patchouly.

Genuine patchouly essential oil has a deep, rich scent. It accurately captures the earthy, musky sweetness of the dried plant. Either form can be used in magical aromatherapy.

The scent of patchouly is useful in arousing sexual desire and has been celebrated as such for well over a century. With proper visualization, it releases anxiety regarding sex and prepares its user for an enjoyable experience.

To get yourself going in the morning, smell patchouly oil for a few seconds. It quickly starts you up.

I'm probably not the only one who's dug up rich, humus-filled dirt and noticed that its scent often closely resembles patchouly. Due to this curious connection, patchouly is also used to manifest needed money. Put a few drops of the dark oil onto a cotton ball. Inhale and visualize.

PENNYROYAL
(Mentha pulegium)

PART USED: fresh or dried leaves
PLANET: Mars
ELEMENT: Fire
MAGICAL INFLUENCES: Physical energy, Conscious mind, Protection

Perhaps as early as 1000 C.E., fresh pennyroyal leaves, mixed with wormwood, were smelled to prevent seasickness during travel.

Sniff the pungent fresh leaves for physical energy, to clear and strengthen the conscious mind and to still dizziness.

The odor is also protective. Inhale with proper visualization.

Warning: Pennyroyal essential oil is extremely hazardous. Do not use.

PEPPERMINT
(Mentha piperita)

PART USED: fresh and dried leaves, essential oil
PLANET: Mercury
ELEMENT: Air
MAGICAL INFLUENCES: Conscious mind, Purification

As long ago as the time of the Roman writer Pliny, the scent of peppermint was used to rouse the conscious mind. It is still powerful for this purpose. The aroma of peppermint also halts negative thoughts, temporarily divorcing you from their effects.

As with most stimulating scents, peppermint should not be used at night unless you don't mind staying up well past your bedtime.

The aroma of peppermint is also useful for self-purification rituals. Inhale with visualization. To purify a room or an entire building, gather fresh bunches of the herb and place in jars of water at various intervals.

PETITGRAIN
(Citrus aurantium)

PART USED: essential oil
PLANET: Sun
ELEMENT: Fire
MAGICAL INFLUENCES: Conscious mind, Protection

Another bitter orange oil, petitgrain is distilled from the leaves of the tree. Its scent is rather harsh with citrusy undertones. Petitgrain bears a resemblance to neroli but lacks its soothing qualities.

Inhale this aroma to ready your conscious mind for further work. Smelling it quickly clears away mental cobwebs, fully awakening you. As with peppermint, this action of petitgrain will often produce a sense of well-being in addition to sharpened thought processes.

The aroma can also be used in conjunction with visualization for personal protection.

PINE
(Pinus sylvestris spp.)

PART USED: fresh pine "needles," essential oil
PLANET: Mars
ELEMENT: Air
MAGICAL INFLUENCES: Healing, Purification, Protection, Physical energy, Magical energy, Money

Walking through a pine forest is an exhilarating experience due to the crisp fragrance drifting on the air.

The aroma of pine speeds healing of the physical body. Inhale often during recuperation (only in conjunction with treatment, of course). Place some in the sickroom as well.

Such a scent is ideal for purification, especially during the winter months. Crush the needles and smell.

Inhale the odor for protection. Visualize all negative energies bearing you as a target being repelled and turned back to their originator(s).

Additionally, the invigorating scent is useful for increasing bioelectrical energy, which is available for magical and physical uses.

And finally, the clean scent of pine is linked with money. Inhale and visualize its scent engendering money-drawing energies. Send these out into the atmosphere to do their work for you.

PLUMERIA
(Plumeria acutifolia)

PART USED: fresh flowers
PLANET: Venus
ELEMENT: Water
MAGICAL INFLUENCES: Peace, Love

The plumeria, native to Mexico, was apparently utilized by the ancient Aztecs in drinks which combatted fear and faintheartedness. If so, this was an extraordinary practice, for the milky sap of the plant is poisonous.

This tree, so at home in the deserts of Mexico, has been extensively planted in Hawaii and the islands of the South Pacific. It is the favorite lei flower.

The scent of plumeria flowers differs from one hybrid to another (there are dozens of forms). However, it commonly has a sweet, lemony fragrance that isn't cloying.

The aroma can be used with visualization to vanquish fear and depression. This promotes a peaceful attitude. Additionally, its fragrance is used to manifest loving relationships.

If you pick the flowers, wipe off the milky sap that accumulates at the base of the blooms.

Unfortunately, no true plumeria essential oil is available, but plants can be found in some nurseries and by mail—see Appendix II.

ROSE
(Rosa damascena)
(Rosa centifolia)

PART USED: fresh flowers, essential oil (otto), absolute

PLANET: Venus

ELEMENT: Water

MAGICAL INFLUENCES: Love, Peace, Sex, Beauty

LORE:

After Europe's "conversion" to the Christian religion, the rose was forbidden to be used as a symbol of the Virgin Mary because of its earlier associations with Venus, Bacchus and other classical deities. A flower with such a past (divine drunkenness, sex and love) was deemed unsuited for the Virgin. Thus, the purer lily was adopted as Her floral symbol.

An incredibly expensive aromatic, rose has a long history of use in cosmetic and magical perfumery. Legend states that it was the first essential oil ever distilled (in Persia during the tenth century). Huge quantities of fresh rose petals are necessary to produce the smallest amount of true essential oil or absolute. This accounts for its price.

Traditionally, rose petals are steam distilled to produce the essential oil known as otto of rose or rose attar. The fragrance is also extracted through the use of solvents to create rose absolute. Of the two, the absolute is considered to be inferior to the otto. It is also less expensive.

Some holistic aromatherapists disdain the use of rose absolute for therapeutic purposes, preferring the true otto of rose. This is partly for health reasons (it's difficult to remove all of the solvent from the oil after processing.) To each their own. Solvent-extracted rose has been used in cosmetic perfumery for some time. I've also used it with no problems.

If you cannot afford these wondrous substances, grow or find the most odorous blooms available. Generally speaking, the darkest roses have the richest scents. Modern hybridizing has all but killed the fragrance of many forms. Most of the roses available from florist shops are virtually scentless.

The following information can be utilized with true rose absolute, otto of rose or with fresh rose flowers. Synthetics should not, of course, be used.

MAGICAL USES:

The first association many of us have with roses is love, and here again modern aromatherapy research supports this timeless link. The scent of roses does indeed turn our thoughts to love. Inhale the deep scent and visualize its energies leading you into a mutually satisfying emotional relationship.

To spread this loving energy throughout your home, place fresh roses in every room. The scent calms domestic strife. Doing this before gatherings ensures a warm, happy time for all who attend. The aroma of roses instills feelings of peace and happiness which are related to love.

Roses are also aphrodisiac, acting directly upon the brain and sexual centers of the body. The fragrance is of immense help in alleviating the sexual problems of women. Inhale the scent and visualize.

It is also helpful in overcoming cases of psychological impotence in men and, as Robert Tisserand writes in *The Art of Aromatherapy*, may increase sperm count.

Women can utilize the scent of roses to enhance their own inner beauty and, hence, their outward appearance. Stand before a mirror with a rose or one sacrificial drop of rose absolute or otto on a cotton ball. Stare into your eyes' reflection. Visualize yourself as a confident, beautiful person. Inhale the mesmerizingly lovely, intensely floral scent.

Allow the rose energy to banish all doubts about your appearance, about your attractiveness. Don't just believe that it can—actually feel it happening. Let the fragrance and the energies work with you in creating your needed change.

Repeat this simple ritual once a day for a week.

ROSEMARY
(Rosemarinus officinalis)

PART USED: fresh or dried leaves, essential oil
PLANET: Sun
ELEMENT: Fire
MAGICAL INFLUENCES: Longevity, Conscious
    mind, Memory, Love
LORE:

Once burned in Greek temples as offerings to the goddesses and gods, rosemary has a long folk magic tradition as a love stimulator. Bridal wreaths were entwined with fresh rosemary and the plant has been used in countless rituals designed to promote love.

Leyel (see Bibliography) records an unusual use of rosemary from an old book:

> "Take the flowers thereof and make pow-
> der thereof and binde it to thy right arme in a lin-
> nen cloath and it shall make *theee* light and
> merrie." (sic)

MAGICAL USES:

Human beings have used rosemary for various magical pursuits for at least 2,500 years. This was due to its clean, resinousy odor and its energies. It currently enjoys great popularity in coventional aromatherapy.

The subtler energies contained with the scent of rosemary are very effective. Here are some of the ways to utilize them:

Smell the scent of rosemary or of its wood while visualizing a long, healthy life, for as an ancient writer put it:

"Smell it oft and it shall keep thee youngly."

Sniff the essential oil or the fresh leaves to clear your conscious mind. Its legendary powers of enhancing the memory, immortalized by William Shakespeare, are genuine. When studying something that you absolutely must memorize, keep the herb or a few drops of rosemary essential oil on a cotton ball beside you. Sniff it often as you study.

Then, when you must recall it (such as during a test or, perhaps, when saying a prayer or chant) smell the essential oil again and the information will make itself available.

As for love, rosemary can help us out there too. Inhale the crisp scent and strongly visualize it bringing love into your life. Carry some with you (or the cotton ball you've used) and smell it a few times throughout the day.

Snips of fresh rosemary are available in the produce sections of some grocery stores, and the essential oil is available at very reasonable prices.

RUE
(Ruta graveolens)

PART USED: fresh leaves
PLANET: Mars
ELEMENT: Fire
MAGICAL INFLUENCES: Calming emotions, Conscious mind, Health

Gerard stated that the juice of rue, when applied to the human body, prevented snakes, spiders, scorpions, bees, hornets and wasps from biting and stinging. It also guarded against poisoning by monkshook (wolf's bane) and fungi.

Many people dislike the powerful scent of rue. I happen to like it, but then I've always valued my non-conformity. Rue is often described as "disagreeable" or "stinking." I can only say that our acceptance or rejection of certain scents is a personal matter.

The biting fragrance of rue calms raging emotions of all kinds: jealousy, depression, love-obsession, anger, hatred, bigotry. The scent eases the pain of broken personal relationships and lessens the ache of non-mutual love. Sniff and push the matter out of your mind.

It powerfully affects the conscious mind, sharpening and fine-tuning it. Rue can also close down access to psychic information. This may seem to be a strange "magical" effect, but some persons are so swamped with psychic information that they can barely lead normal lives. Rue is one answer to this rare but difficult problem.

Sniff fresh rue once a day or so (if you have access to the herb) to maintain good health.

Warning: The essential oil is extremely hazardous and should not be used. Even simple handling of the fresh herb itself may cause allergic reactions in some individuals. Be careful.

SAFFRON
(Crocus sativus)
PART USED: dried stigmas
PLANET: Sun
ELEMENT: Fire

MAGICAL INFLUENCES Conscious mind, Physical
    energy, Magical energy, Money
LORE:

A sacred flower in ancient Crete, saffron has a
long history of religious and magical use. Greek goddesses and gods wore robes dyed with saffron, as did
Buddhist monks. At one point in ancient Greece,
saffron-colored clothing was a distinctive badge of the
nobility as well as of prostitutes

Robert Tisserand writes in *Aromatherapy for Everyone*
that saffron may have been an ingredient in the famous
Egyptian incense *kyphi* (see Chapter 2 of this book). In
Rome, saffron was burned with frankincense, myrrh
and other costly rarities in honor of the deities. The
Phoenicians baked it into cakes which were offered to
Ashtoreth, the goddess of the Moon. They also ate
them to induce human fertility.

Early Persian women called upon saffron to
ensure speedy childbirth. The men used it to raise the
winds. Around 1600, saffron oil was rubbed onto the
forehead to prevent drunkenness. And lizards are
said to detest the scent so much that they stay away
from any place that contains saffron.

It is an ancient symbol of the Sun and has long
been used to give certain foods (such as rice and
bread) a distinctive yellow color which is connected
with solar worship.

Don't confuse this with the Mexican culinary
spice *Azafran*. Genuine saffron is currently the most
expensive spice still being traded. I recently purchased
two small samples of saffron. The first, weighing in at
0.008 oz. (eight hundredths of an ounce) set me back
only $2.95, while 0.06 oz. (1.7 grams) of saffron cost

about 11 dollars. It is available at some herb and gourmet cooking shops.

Saffron has a long, gilded history. During the
Middle Ages, a pound or so of the bulbs from which
the flowers sprout were accepted as security for loans
just as were gold and jewelry. In Nuremburg in 1444
and 1456, people were burned alive for adulterating
saffron.

A curious fact: the English town of Saffron-Walden
was once known for growing the flower there. The
fields are long gone but the C. W. Daniel publishing
company, which produces books on aromatherapy, is
located in Saffron-Walden.

But what is saffron? The spice consists of the
dried red and yellow stigmas of the flowers. They're
so light that about 4,320 flowers (figures vary) yield
only one ounce of saffron.

All this background information should put us in
the proper frame of mind to utilize the evocative scent
of saffron in magical aromatherapy.

MAGICAL USES:

It possesses a warm, stimulating aroma unlike
any other. Smell it first thing in the morning to kick-
start your body, to energize yourself. Saffron makes a
wonderful prep for the day's activities.

The scent awakens the conscious mind and sharpens mental alertness. Inhale the fragrance prior to
magical ritual for expanded bioelectrical energy.
Visualize as you do this, perhaps seeing the scent as
threads of burnished, golden light pouring into your
body.

Saffron has long been associated with gold. Its

high price and scarcity also account for its use in manifesting increased money. Sniff and visualize prosperity coming into your life.

The ancient writers rhapsodized about the scent of saffron which, to be truthful, is distinctive but rather scant. It is odd that the British herbalist Culpeper warned that overindulgence of this fragrance had led to "immoderate convulsive laughter, which ended in death." Perhaps this was a reaction to the outrageous price of this beautiful spice.

SAGE
(Salvia officinalis)

PART USED: fresh leaves, dried leaves
PLANET: Juniper
ELEMENT: Air
MAGICAL INFLUENCES: Memory, Conscious mind, Wisdom, Money

The leaves of this common culinary herb possess such a strong, heady scent that they have long been used in magic. American Indians utilized white sage and other species of this fragrant plant in religious rituals.

Since at least the 16th century, sage has been sniffed to strengthen the ability to memorize and to tone the conscious mind. With visualization it can also be used to promote wisdom.

European folk magicians use sage as a bringer of money. Crush fresh or dried sage leaves between your fingers. Visualize money coming into your life or, if desired, those things which money will bring to you. See them manifesting in your life.

Warning: Sage essential oil contains high levels of the

ketone *thujone*, a dangerous substance. It should not be used at all, particularly by pregnant women. The fresh or dried herb is safe for use.

SANDALWOOD
(Santalum album)

PART USED: wood, essential oil
PLANET: Moon
ELEMENT: Water
MAGICAL INFLUENCES Spirituality, Meditation, Sex, Healing
LORE:

The word is not derived from "sandal" but from the Sanskrit *chandana*.

Sandalwood is commercially grown only in India, where every tree is numbered and protected by the government. Various wild species of sandalwood can be found on many Pacific islands, including the Hawaiian chain.

The woodsy, warm, rather astringent scent of this wood has long been used as incense by the Chinese. In India, temples built solely of sandalwood centuries ago are said to still emit the odor of this wood, and in Hawaii some early missionary houses were constructed with beams of sandalwood.

When early traders discovered this fragrant wood in Hawaii, they began the tortuous sandalwood trade, forcing the local Hawaiian population to turn from subsistence farming to gathering sandalwood. The effects were so devastating that some Hawaiians pulled up young trees to prevent their descendants from suffering the same fate. Isolated stands of sandalwood trees can still be found there, but their exact locations are kept secret from outsiders.

MAGICAL USES:

Thousands of years ago, the scent of sandalwood was discovered to induce spirituality and the peace of religious union. Its soothing aroma lulls the conscious mind and prepares us for rituals of all kinds. Inhaling the fragrance of sandalwood or its essential oil prior to religious rituals and meditation creates the proper mood.

Visualizing accordingly, the aroma of sandalwood is also useful in stimulating sexual activity. It has been termed one of the true aphrodisiacs. In cases of emotional or mental sexual dysfunction (frigidity, impotency), sandalwood can effect a cure.

To speed healing, add a few drops of sandalwood essential oil to your bath water and visualize its scent and energies doing their work.

Because sandalwood essential oil is somewhat expensive, the wood can be substituted. Search for good quality wood. Sawdust and small chips are available in this country. These are byproducts of the sandalwood carving industry in India. If a friend is traveling to Hong Kong, have them bring you back small chunks of the wood, which can be easily found.

In Asian stores, metaphysical shops and Eastern mysticism centers, look for sandalwood beads, carved elephants and other objects made from this wood. All are useful for these purposes.

SPEARMINT
(Mentha spicata)

PART USED: fresh leaves, essential oil
PLANET: Mercury

ELEMENT: Air
MAGICAL INFLUENCES: Healing, Protection during sleep

The fresh scent of spearmint is inhaled with visualization to speed healing of the body. Use the fragrance to key into your bioelectrical energy, redirecting it toward the healing process.

At night, place fresh sprigs of this aromatic plant in your bedroom or fill a small bag with spearmint and lay it on your pillow. Inhale its scent as you fall asleep, visualizing it wrapping you with protective energy.

The odor of spearmint is also refreshing and comforting to the bereaved.

SPIDER LILY
(Hymenocallis littoralis)

PART USED: fresh flowers
PLANET: Venus
ELEMENT: Water
MAGICAL INFLUENCES: Love, Peace

I woke before dawn on my first morning on the Hawaiian island of Kauai. Stumbling to my hotel room's double glass doors, I looked outside. Rain splattered down, rustling the coconut palms and luxuriant foliage. I opened the door and walked into the moist air.

Just outside was a stand of spider lilies, their six-pointed, petal-drooping flowers dancing in the rainfall. I bent toward them and inhaled the sweet, luxuriant scent, forever linking it with the magical place to which I'd gone.

Spider lily plants are available in mainland nurseries. Sniff the flowers while visualizing love, or let the sweet fragrance soak into you, calming strife and creating peace.

Unfortunately, there is no true essential oil.

STAR ANISE
(Illicum verum)

PART USED: dried fruit
PLANET: Jupiter
ELEMENT: Air
MAGICAL INFLUENCES: Psychic awareness

A related species of this tree is often planted near Buddhist temples. In Japan, the bark is used as incense.

The fruit resembles an eight-pointed star. Each point contains a shiny brown seed. Star anise emits a powerful licorice-like odor.

It is this fragrance which is useful for enhancing psychic awareness. Inhale the scent while sitting quietly. Still your conscious mind. Allow the star anise energy to enter you, soothing your conscious mind and awakening your submerged psychic abilities.

STEPHANOTIS
(Stephanotis floribunda)

PART USED: fresh flowers
PLANET: Moon
ELEMENT: Water
MAGICAL INFLUENCES: Love, Peace

A traditional wedding flower, stephanotis is often included in bridal bouquets. It is native to Madagascar but is usually associated with Hawaii.

The sweet, delicate scent of these throated white

flowers promotes love for ourselves and for others. Because of their connection with weddings, stephanotis blossoms can be sniffed to ease the often stormy sea of matrimony.

The fragrance also instills peace and happiness.

Though the cut flowers are expensive (when available) and no true stephanotis essential oil is sold, the plant can be grown indoors or, in temperate climates, outdoors.

SWEET PEA
(Lathrys odoratus)

PART USED: fresh flowers
PLANET: Mercury
ELEMENT: Air
MAGICAL INFLUENCES: Happiness, Courage

No true sweet pea essential oil is available, so the fresh flowers must be used. But they're so beautiful and smell so sweet that this is no great strain.

Sniff the flowers to uplift yourself, to transport your consciousness to a slightly higher rung of awareness. The flowers themselves look so cheery that it's not surprising their fragrance promotes this state within human beings.

Also, with visualization, inhale the delicate scent to gently incline yourself to courage and strength in the face of depression or great adversity. Smell before employment interviews or stressful social situations. Sniff and let the aroma of sweet pea instill confidence within you.

The seeds are available in garden shops everywhere, and some varieties do nicely in small pots. Plant for spring blooms.

THYME

(Thymus vulgaris)

PART USED: fresh leaves and flowers
PLANET: Venus
ELEMENT: Water
MAGICAL INFLUENCES: Courage, Conscious mind,
    Health

Our word thyme was derived from the Greek word
for perfuming, *thymos*. This is fitting, for the tiny
leaves emit a powerful scent. Thyme was burned in
ancient temples. The Roman naturalist Pliny stated
that when burned, thyme drove off all venomous
creatures.

The fragrance has long been known to promote
courage and so can be inhaled with visualization for
this purpose.

To stimulate the conscious mind, simply smell its
sharp scent. This may explain why placing thyme
under the pillow is thought to prevent nightmares.
The scent shuts down the psychic mind (which often
produces dreams). But by its stimulating action on
the conscious mind, thyme may prevent sleep, which
certainly prevents all dreams—positive or negative.

Thyme is also called upon to maintain good health.
Smell it once a day with visualization, allowing its
energies to revitalize your body.

Warning: *The Essential Oil Safety Data Manual* states
that thyme essential oil is only slightly less toxic than
sage. It should not be used, especially by pregnant
women.

TONKA

(Dipteryx odorata)

PART USED: The dried, cured seeds ("beans")
PLANET: Jupiter
ELEMENT: Earth
MAGICAL INFLUENCES: Money

Until recently, many U.S. citizens bought "vainilla" in Tijuana, thinking they were buying genuine vanilla extract. Instead, they were picking up the extract of this plant. As long ago as 1931 (Grieve; see Bibliography) it was known that large doses of tonka dangerously affected the heart. Recently, tonka "vainilla" was banned for importation to the U.S., but is still sold in Mexico.

Because of this recent scare, tonka "beans" were suddenly hard to find and are extremely expensive. However, some potpourri supply stores still stock them.

The seeds contain large amounts of coumarin, which is a vanilla-like substance found in many other plants such as deerstongue and woodruff.

The plant wasn't named for the famous toy trucks.

In magical aromatherapy, the fragrance of tonka beans can be inhaled with visualization to manifest needed money. Do this no more than once or twice a week and don't lick the seeds!

Warning: Keep out of the reach of children, who may mistake the fragrant black seeds for candy.

TUBEROSE
(Polianthes tuberosa)

PART USED: fresh flowers
PLANET: Venus
ELEMENT: Water
MAGICAL INFLUENCES: Peace, Love

This plant is native to Mexico. Under the name of *omixochitl*, it was used by the Aztec herbalists for treating various complaints. *Omixochitl* means "bone-flower," from the whiteness of its flowers that, to them, must have resembled bones.

True tuberose essential oil is produced by *enfleurage*, the most expensive method. This substance is costly and rarely available at the retail level. It is used in such cosmetic perfumes as White Shoulders.

This plant's flowers are similar to jasmine in that they continue to produce scent even after being picked. The fragrance is much stronger at night than during the day. Because of this, tuberose is known in India as *rat ki rani* (mistress of the night).

The waxy, white blooms are intensely fragrant, sweet but not cloying. The cut flowers are available in florist shops on the West Coast and are apparently gaining in popularity. The bulbs may be purchased from nurseries and cultivated for their blooms.

Like many people, my first run-in with this plant was in the Honolulu International Airport, where thousands of tuberose leis are given to arriving tourists. The scent is so strong that it permeates the air there.

The scent of fresh tuberose stills raging passions, calms and soothes the emotions. Smell the flowers to gain control.

With visualization, the aroma of tuberose invites love into your life or expands the love you're already enjoying.

TULIP
(*Tulipa* spp.)
PART USED: fresh flowers
PLANET: Venus
ELEMENT: Earth
MAGICAL INFLUENCES: Purification

Many people seem unaware that tulips are scented, but most varieties of this popular bulb plant do emit a soft, sweet but somewhat antiseptic fragrance. Inhale the light odor of the fresh flowers during personal purification rituals.

VANILLA
(*Vanilla planiflora*)
PART USED: the dried, cured fruits ("beans")
PLANET: Venus
ELEMENT: Water
MAGICAL INFLUENCES: Sex, Love, Physical energy, Magical energy
LORE:
   The vanilla "bean" is the product of a native Mexican orchid. A goddess of the vanilla plant was once worshipped there. In American folk magic, women place a few drops of vanilla tincture behind their ears to attract men.

MAGICAL USES:
   The flavor and scent is familiar due to its use in everything from natural cream sodas to cakes and ice

cream. Vanilla extract, so available on grocery store shelves, shouldn't be used for magical aromatherapy. Buy a whole vanilla "bean" for a few dollars (or the absolute, if you can find it and are willing to pay the price).

The warm aroma of vanilla produces sexual arousal when sniffed with proper visualization. More broadly, it can be inhaled to manifest a loving sexual relationship. The sensual fragrance appeals equally to both men and women.

The fragrance of vanilla revitalizes the body, producing bioelectrical energy which can be channeled into physical exertion or magical rituals. Sniff prior to making the extra effort.

VETIVERT
(Vetiveria zizanoides)
AKA: "Vetiver," "Khus Khus"

PART USED: the dried, ground rootstock; the essential oil
PLANET: Venus
ELEMENT: Earth
MAGICAL INFLUENCES: Protection, Money

The scent of vetivert is woodsy, strong and uplifting. The root is extensively used in folk magic for both protection and money, and its aroma has the same effects.

To guard yourself, inhale the fragrance while visualizing it sealing your body from negative energies. For home protection, place a few drops of the essential oil into a diffusor or potpourri simmerer and visualize.

Vetivert is ideal for manifesting increased money in your life. Simply visualize this needed change while sniffing its rich aroma. Repeat as necessary.

Some import stores offer fans fashioned of woven vetivert roots. Look for them.

WATER LILY
(Nymphaea coerula or *Nymphaea* spp.)
PART USED: fresh flowers
PLANET: Moon
ELEMENT: Water
MAGICAL INFLUENCES: Peace, Happiness, Love
LORE:

Virtually every book written about ancient Egypt has described that fabled peoples' love affair with the "lotus." Representations of it abound. One memorable image: a carving of Tutankhamen as a newborn child emerging from a lotus flower.

As mentioned in Chapter 2 of this book, overwhelming evidence now indicates that the true lotus *(Nelumbo nucifera)* was unknown in Egypt until its fairly late introduction by the Persians. The flower that the Egyptians loved, treasured and worshipped above all others was actually the water lily.

It was the water lily that graced the rectangular garden pools. It was the water lily that was associated with Ra, Isis and Osiris. The true lotus, of Indian origin, is an entirely different plant as can be observed when comparing traditional Indian paintings of the lotus with Egyptian art.

MAGICAL USES:

It's rather hard to smell a fresh water lily blossom. Such a feat may entail wading through water. Here in southern California, many people raise them in backyard pools but the cut flowers are never available.

However, no book about fragrance could ignore this famous aroma.

The blue water lily emits a pleasingly sweet scent (the botanical building in Balboa Park, in San Diego, has a koi pool fringed with water lilies and real loti). In ancient Egypt, it was found to produce a peaceful disposition and to create happiness, which is why the flower was smelled at celebrations and feasts.

Additionally, the scent of the water lily can be inhaled with visualization to manifest a loving relationship.

No true lotus or water lily essential oils are available.

WOOD ALOE
(Aquilaria agallocha)

PART USED: dried wood
PLANET: Venus
ELEMENT: Water
MAGICAL INFLUENCES: Spirituality, Meditation, Love

Wood aloe, which is finally appearing on the American retail herb market, is a richly-scented wood long used for medicinal and religious purposes in China and Japan. Some people may find the fragrance too strong but I like it. It smells of ancient temples, ancient magic, of power and spirituality.

Inhale the deep aroma of wood aloe to create a heightened state of spirituality. This is an evocative introduction to religious rituals of all kinds. The fragrance also heightens meditation.

Sniff the aroma of the wood, with visualization, to bring you to someone who's looking for a loving relationship.

WOODRUFF
(Asperula odorata)
PART USED: fresh and dried leaves
PLANET: Mars
ELEMENT: Fire
MAGICAL INFLUENCES: Purification, Success

Woodruff has been used in European folk magic since at least 1000 C.E. It is well known as a flavoring ingredient in May Wine, a traditional drink of May 1st.

The plant emits a warm, vanilla-like odor but doesn't possess the same properties as do other plants which produce this aroma (such as deerstongue and tonka). The fragrance is inhaled with visualization for internal spiritual purification. One side effect of such a ritual may be a feeling of peace and happiness.

Due to its usage in folk magic, the scent is also inhaled in conjunction with the proper visualizations to ensure success in all pursuits.

YARROW
(Achillea millefolium)
PART USED: fresh flowers, dried flowers, essential oil
PLANET: Venus
ELEMENT: Water
MAGICAL INFLUENCES: Psychic awareness, Courage, Love

These flowers produce a rich, full-bodied scent. The essential oil is a beautiful blue due to its azulene content. Its aroma is even more astonishing. Yarrow essential oil is also, unfortunately, expensive.

Yarrow is an excellent choice for those wishing to hone their psychic awareness. The aroma, when sniffed with visualization, lulls the conscious mind and allows true psychic communicataion to take place. Place a few drops onto a cotton ball, hold it up to your nose and inhale while in a relaxed sitting position.

For a far different purpose, smell the flowers to instill courage within yourself. Do this, of course, with proper visualization.

Yarrow has been a part of love charms for countless centuries. The scent magnifies love for self and for others, and so can be utilized in love-attracting rituals.

YLANG-YLANG
(Canaga odorata)

PART USED: essential oil
PLANET: Venus
ELEMENT: Water
MAGICAL INFLUENCES: Peace, Sex, Love

In his recent book (*Aromatherapy for Everyone*), Robert Tisserand recorded an alleged instance in which the aroma of ylang-ylang essential oil calmed a vicious dog seconds before it attacked a man.

The flowers from which ylang-ylang essential oil is produced are as exotic as their name and scent. The tree is grown far away on sun-drenched islands such as the Philippines, Java and Sumatra. A few trees may be seen growing in Florida and Hawaii.

Ylang-ylang is a soothing scent. Wear it or inhale its aroma prior to all nerve-wracking situations such as job interviews. Smell its sweet, incredible fragrance.

Simultaneously, breathe in its soothing energies and visualize them doing their work. You'll get through just fine.

The fragrance also calms anger and all negative emotional states, transforming such energy into more positive manifestations. It inclines to rest, comfort, and sleep.

With proper visualization it is also a powerful, true aphrodisiac, creating sexual desire. As with all essential oils of this kind, sniff the fragrance with specific visualization. Ylang-ylang is exceptionally helpful in overcoming sexual problems.

Ylang-ylang is also used for love.

Patricia Davis, in her excellent *Aromatherapy: An A-Z*, writes that inhaling this essential oil for long periods of time can produce headache and/or nausea. I've never found this to be true but perhaps I know when to stop.

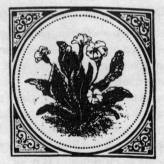

PART III

TABLES

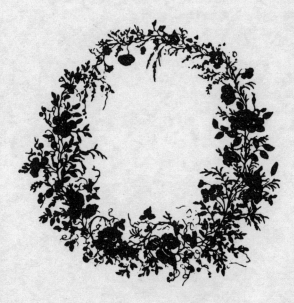

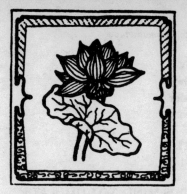

These tables summarize some of the information included in Part II of this book. Additional tables of ritual correspondences are also listed here for use as intuition dictates. For information not included here, see the index.

Remember, these tables include fresh and dried plant materials as well as essential oils. Those marked with an * should *not* be used in essential oil form!

MAGICAL CHANGES AND RECOMMENDED SCENTS/ESSENTIAL OILS

Please see Part II for explicit information regarding usage of these scents.

APHRODISIAC. See SEX

ASTRAL PROJECTION
   *Mugwort

BEAUTY, TO ENHANCE
   Catnip
   Rose

CELIBACY
Camphor
Lavender
*Marjoram

COMFORT
Calendula

CONSCIOUS MIND, TO STIMULATE

*Basil
Bay
Black Pepper
Caraway
Coffee
Costmary
Dill
*Hyssop
Lavender
Lily of the Valley
*Pennyroyal
Peppermint
Rosemary
*Rue
Saffron
*Sage
*Thyme

COURAGE

Black Pepper
Clove
Fennel
Ginger
Onion
Sweet Pea
*Thyme
Yarrow

DEPRESSION, TO RELIEVE

*Basil
Clary Sage
Jasmine
*Lemon Balm
*Ylang-Ylang

DREAMS, PSYCHIC

Calendula
Jasmine
Mimosa
*Mugwort

DREAMS, VIVID
Clary Sage

EMOTIONS, STILLING
Costmary
*Rue

EUPHORIA
Clary Sage

HAPPINESS/JOY

Apple	Neroli
*Basil	Sweet Pea
Bergamot	Water Lily
Orange	

HEALING

Clove	Myrrh
Coriander	Niaouli
Cypress	Palmarosa
Eucalyptus	Pine
Hops	Sandalwood
Melon	Spearmint

HEALTH, TO MAINTAIN

Carnation	Melon
Eucalyptus	Pine
Garlic	*Rue
Lavender	*Thyme
Lemon	

LONGEVITY
    Fennel
    Rosemary

LOVE

Apple	Meadowsweet
Cardamon	Mimosa
Carnation	Narcissus
Coriander	Palmarosa
Daffodil	Plumeria
Freesia	Rose
Gardenia	Rosemary
Ginger	Spider Lily
Ginger, White	Stephanotis
Hyacinth	Tuberose
Iris	Vanilla
Jasmine	Water Lily
Lavender	Wood Aloe
Lemon Verbena	Yarrow
Lilac	Ylang-Ylang

MAGICAL ENERGY

Bay	Nutmeg
Carnation	Orange
Galangal	Pine
Ginger	Vanilla

MEDITATION

Camomile	Sandalwood
Frankincense	Wood Aloe
Myrrh	

MEMORY
  Clove   Rosemary
  Coriander   *Sage
  Lily of the Valley

MONEY
  *Basil   Patchouly
  Ginger   *Sage
  Lemon Balm   Tonka
  Nutmeg   Vetivert
  Oak Moss

PEACE
  Apple   Lily
  Bergamot   Lily of the Valley
  Broom   *Marjoram
  Camomile   Meadowsweet
  Catnip   Plumeria
  Freesia   Rose
  Gardenia   Spider Lily
  Ginger, White   Stephanotis
  Jasmine   Tuberose
  Lavender   Water Lily
  Lemon Balm   Ylang-ylang

PHYSICAL ENERGY
  Bay   Garlic
  Bergamot Mint   Ginger
  Black Pepper   Lemon
  Camphor   Lime
  Caraway   Nasturtium
  Carnation   Nutmeg
  Cinnamon   Orange

PHYSICAL ENERGY (continued)

Patchouly
*Pennyroyal
Pine

Saffron
Vanilla

PROSPERITY

Bergamot Mint
Cinnamon

Honeysuckle
SEE ALSO Money

PROTECTION

*Basil
Black Pepper
Broom
Clove
Cumin
Galangal
Garlic
Geranium
Juniper

Lime
Nasturtium
Niaouli
Onion
Parsley
Peppermint
*Pennyroyal
Pine
Vetivert

PSYCHIC AWARENESS

Bay
Celery
Cereus, Night-Blooming
Cinnamon
Deerstongue
Iris

Lemongrass
Mace
*Mugwort
Nutmeg
Star Anise
Yarrow

PURIFICATION

Bay
Broom
Camphor
Copal

Costmary
Dill
Eucalyptus
Garlic

PURIFICATION (continued)

Ginger, White	Lilac
*Hyssop	Lime
Juniper	Neroli
Lemon	Orange
Lemon Balm	Pine
Lemongrass	Tulip
Lemon Verbena	Wood Aloe

SEX (Aphrodisiacs)

Cardamon	Rose
Ginger	Sandalwood
Jasmine	Vanilla
Neroli	Ylang-Ylang
Patchouly	

SEX (Anaphrodisiacs)
Camphor
*Marjoram
SEE ALSO Celibacy

SLEEP

Bergamot	Hyacinth
Camomile	Jasmine
Celery	Lavender
Hops	*Marjoram

SLEEP, PROTECTION DURING
Spearmint

SPIRITUALITY

Cedar	Myrrh
Frankincense	Sandalwood
Gardenia	Wood Aloe
Jasmine	

SUCCESS
   Woodruff

WEIGHT LOSS
   Honeysuckle

WISDOM
   *Sage

AROMAS OF THE DAYS OF THE WEEK

Check this list (or compose your own) for essential oils and plants linked with each day. These may be used for daily rituals. Aromas have been recommended according to the planetary ruler of the days of the week.

MONDAY (Moon): Jasmine, Lemon, Sandalwood, Stephanotis

TUESDAY (Mars): *Basil, Coriander, Ginger, Nasturtium

WEDNESDAY (Mercury): Benzoin, Clary Sage, Eucalyptus, Lavender

THURSDAY (Jupiter): Clove, Lemon Balm (Melissa), Oakmoss, Star Anise

FRIDAY (Venus): Cardamom, Palmarosa, Rose, Yarrow

SATURDAY (Saturn): Cypress, Mimosa, Myrrh, Patchouly

SUNDAY (Sun): Cedar, Frankincense, Neroli, Rosemary

AROMAS OF THE SEASONS

Use these aromas (plants or essential oils) to welcome each new season in personal ritual observances.

SPRING: Daffodil, Jasmine, Rose; all sweet scents
SUMMER: Carnation, Clove, Ginger; all spicy scents
AUTUMN: Oakmoss, Patchouly, Vetivert; all earthy scents
WINTER: Frankincense, Pine, Rosemary; all resinous scents

AROMAS OF THE LUNAR CYCLES

FIRST QUARTER: Sandalwood
FULL MOON: Jasmine
LAST QUARTER: Lemon
NEW MOON: Camphor

Inhale these aromas during the phases of the Moon to attune with lunar energy. Sandalwood, appropriate for the First Quarter and the Moon's waxing, enhances spirituality. Jasmine possesses the full-blown energies of the Full Moon. The more ethereal lemon is symbolic of the lessening of the Moon's influence as She wanes (Last Quarter) while the coldness of camphor signifies the similarly cold New Moon.

AFFINITIES OF ESSENTIAL OILS
WITH CRYSTALS

This is a short list of recommended stones for use in conjunction with essential oils during magical rituals. Use your imagination in discovering ways in which to do this. For example, hold the stone and visualize its energy entering your body through your palm. Inhale the essential oil, adding its force to your programmed bioelectrical energy. Retain this energy for an internal change or send it out for an external change. Place one drop of the essential oil onto the stone and carry it with you.

There are numerous other methods. Experiment and find what works best for you.

BLACK PEPPER: Bloodstone. Courage, physical energy.

CARDAMOM: Carnelian. Sex, overcoming sexual dysfunction.

CEDARWOOD: Lepidolite. Spirituality, sleep, proection.

EUCALYPTUS: Aquamarine. Health, healing, purification.

FRANKINCENSE: Amber. Strength, healing, protection.

GERANIUM: Red Tourmaline. Protection.

GINGER: Rhodochrosite. Physical energy, love.

JASMINE: Moonstone. Love, sleep, psychic awareness.

JUNIPER: Red Jasper. Protection.

LAVENDER: Fluorite. Healing, health, conscious mind.

NEROLI: Chrysoprase. Happiness, joy.

NIAOULI: Imperial Topaz. Protection.

PALMAROSA: Lapis Lazuli. Love, healing.

PATCHOULY: Green Tourmaline. Money.

PINE: Malachite. Magical energy, money, protection.

ROSE: Rose Quartz. Love, peace, happiness.

ROSEMARY: Quartz Crystal. All *positive* magical changes.

SANDALWOOD: Clear Calcite. Spirituality, meditation.

YARROW: Amethyst. Love, psychic awareness.

YLANG-YLANG: Kunzite. Love, peace.

AROMAS OF THE ELEMENTS

In traditional magical teachings, the elements are emanations from the one source of energy that created the universe, known by the Sanskrit word *Akasha*. Each of the four elements (Earth, Air, Fire, Water) possesses its own distinct energies that are useful in magic. In brief, these energies are:

EARTH: Money, businesses, material objects, foundation, conservation, ecology, grounding

AIR: Conscious mind, mentation, movement, travel, communication, teaching, overcoming addictions.

FIRE: Sex, breaking habits, purification, protection,

banishing illness, aggression, health, strength
WATER: Love, purification, psychic awareness, healing, friendships, beauty, spirituality, meditation

The following table summarizes the elemental attributions given to each plant and essential oil in this book. This is a personal system I've developed during the last 18 years. It is constantly evolving as I gain new insights into the energies contained within plants. Other books contain different attributions. None are incorrect; all are correct to their respective users. Create your own correspondences if these don't speak to you.

EARTH: Cypress, Honeysuckle, Lilac, Mimosa, Oak-moss, Patchouly, Tonka, Tulip, Vetivert
AIR: Bergamot Mint, Caraway, Celery, Clary Sage, Costmary, Dill, Eucalyptus, Fennel, Hops, Lavender, Lemon Balm, Lemongrass, Lemon Verbena, Lily of the Valley, *Marjoram, Meadowsweet, Niaouli, Parsley, Peppermint, Pine, *Sage, Spearmint, Star Anise, Sweet Pea
FIRE: *Basil, Bay, Bergamot, Black Pepper, Broom, Calendula, Carnation, Clove, Coffee, Copal, Coriander, Cumin, Deerstongue, Frankincense, Galangal, Garlic, Ginger, *Hyssop, Juniper, Lime, Nasturtium, Neroli, Nutmeg, Onion, Orange, *Pennyroyal, Petitgrain, Rosemary, *Rue, Saffron, Woodruff
WATER: Apple, Camomile, Camphor, Cardamom, Freesia, Gardenia, Geranium, Hyacinth, Iris, Jasmine, Lemon, Lily, Magnolia, Melon, *Mugwort, Myrrh, Narcissus, Night-Blooming Cereus, Palma-

rosa, Plumeria, Rose, Sandalwood, Spider Lily, Stephanotis, *Thyme, Vanilla, Water Lily, White Ginger, Wood Aloe, Yarrow, Ylang-Ylang

AROMAS OF THE PLANETS

Like the elements, the seven planets known to ancient peoples were linked with plants and scents. The Sun and Moon were included along with Mercury, Venus, Mars, Jupiter and Saturn as planets, and, in spite of modern astronomical knowledge, this system has been retained in many forms of folk magic. The general magical energies of the planets are:

SUN: protection, healing, success, magical power, physical energy

MOON: psychic awareness, psychic dreams, sleep, love, healing, fertility, peace, compassion, spirituality, meditation

MERCURY: intelligence, conscious mind, eloquence, study, self-improvement, overcoming addictions, breaking habits, travel, communication

VENUS: love, fidelity, reconciliation, beauty, youth, joy and happiness, friendships

MARS: aggression, courage, healing after surgery, physical strength, politics, sexual energy, protection, defense, physical energy, magical energy

JUPITER: materialism, money, prosperity, foundation, expansion.

SATURN: purification, longevity, finding a new house, money (through Saturn's link with the element of Earth)

As mentioned above, the below lists, summarizing the planetary attributions in this book, are open to change if you feel the need. I've certainly changed them several times. I attribute jasmine to the Moon here. In my first herb book, *Magical Herbalism*, I assigned Jupiter as its ruler. This is just an example of how systems change with time. Once again, neither attribution is correct; this is simply my latest.

SUN: Bay, Bergamot, Calendula, Carnation, Cedar, Cinnamon, Copal, Frankincense, Juniper, Lime, Neroli, Orange, Petitgrain, Rosemary, Saffron

MOON: Camphor, Jasmine, Lemon, Lily, Melon, Night-Blooming Cereus, Sandalwood, Stephanotis, Water Lily

MERCURY: Benzoin, Bergamot Mint, Caraway, Celery, Clary Sage, Costmary, Dill, Eucalyptus, *Fennel, Lavender, Lemon Verbena, Lily of the Valley, *Marjoram, Niaouli, Parsley, Peppermint, Spearmint, Sweet Pea

VENUS: Apple, Camomile, Cardamom, Catnip, Daffodil, Freesia, Gardenia, Geranium, Hyacinth, Iris, Lilac, Magnolia, *Mugwort, Narcissus, Palmarosa, Plumeria, Rose, Spider Lily, *Thyme, Tuberose, Tulip, Vanilla, Vetivert, White Ginger, Wood Aloe, Yarrow, Ylang-Ylang

MARS: *Basil, Black Pepper, Broom, Coffee, Coriander, Cumin, Deerstongue, Galangal, Garlic, Ginger, Hops, Nasturtium Onion, *Pennyroyal, Pine, *Rue, Woodruff

JUPITER: Clove, Honeysuckle, Hyssop, Lemon Balm, Mace, Meadowsweet, Nutmeg, Oakmoss, *Sage, Star Anise, Tonka

SATURN: Cypress, Mimosa, Myrrh, Patchouly

AROMAS OF THE ZODIAC

These are suggested plants and essential oils associated with the signs of the Zodiac. Authorities can't seem to agree on suitable plants for each sign. One important note: regularly utilize such scents *only* if you wish to strengthen your Sun sign's influence in your life. For instance, if you're a Leo and are trying to take the edge off your, say, aggressive nature, constantly sniffing ginger oil would only serve to increase your aggression, unless you specifically visualized otherwise.

Many aromas are listed under more than one sign because of their traditional relationships to the planets and/or elements associated with them. Most planets and the elements rule more than one sign.

ARIES: Black Pepper, Clove, Coriander, Cumin, Frankincense, Ginger, Neroli, *Pennyroyal, Petitgrain, Pine, Woodruff

TAURUS: Apple, Cardamom, Honeysuckle, Lilac, Magnolia, Oakmoss, Patchouly, Plumeria, Rose, *Thyme, Tonka, Ylang-Ylang

GEMINI: Benzoin, Bergamot Mint, Caraway, Dill, Lavender, Lemongrass, Lily of the Valley, Peppermint, Sweet Pea

CANCER (MOON CHILDREN): Camomile, Cardamom, Jasmine, Lemon, Lily, Myrrh, Palmarosa, Plumeria, Rose, Sandalwood, Yarrow

LEO: Bay, *Basil, Cinnamon, Frankincense, Ginger, Juniper, Lime, Nasturtium, Neroli, Orange, Petitgrain, Rosemary

VIRGO: Caraway, Clary Sage, Costmary, Cypress, Dill, Fennel, Lemon Balm, Honeysuckle, Oakmoss, Patchouly

LIBRA: Camomile, Daffodil, Dill, Eucalyptus, Fennel, Geranium, Peppermint, Pine, Spearmint, Palmarosa, Vanilla

SCORPIO: Black Pepper, Cardamom, Coffee, Galangal, Hyacinth. Hops, *Pennyroyal, Pine, *Thyme, Tuberose, Woodruff

SAGITTARIUS: Bergamot, Calendula, Clove, *Hyssop, Lemon Balm, Mace, *Nutmeg, Oakmoss, Rosemary, Saffron

CAPRICORN: Cypress, Honeysuckle, Lilac, Mimosa, Myrrh, Patchouly, Tonka, Tulip, Vetivert

AQUARIUS: Costmary, Hops, Lavender, Lemon Verbena, Parsley, Patchouly, Pine, Star Anise, Sweet Pea

PISCES: Apple, Camphor, Cardamom, Gardenia, Hyacinth, Jasmine, Lily, *Mugwort, Myrrh, Palmarosa, Sandalwood, Vanilla, Ylang-Ylang

ESSENTIAL OIL BLENDS

As mentioned earlier, many of the so-called magical oils sold today are composed of synthetics. Their effectiveness, if any, seems to stem from the psychological impact of the oil's name—not scent.

Blends containing true essential oils are more effective for the reasons I've stated in this book. This section is a short introduction to creating your own genuine magical oils.*

---

* For more information see *The Complete Book of Incense, Oils and Brews* (Scott Cunningham, Llewellyn, 1989).

The Base Oil

Any of the following oils can be used:

Almond	Olive
Apricot kernel	Palm
Grapeseed	Safflower
Hazelnut	Sesame
Jojoba	Sunflower

For best results, use a lightly-scented oil such as jojoba or safflower. For all base oils except jojoba, add a few drops of wheat germ oil before blending. This will help preserve the final product, for essential oils rapidly oxidize once they've been added to the base oil, and the base itself will become rancid. The only exception to this is jojoba oil, which is pressed from the fruits of the jojoba plant (*Simmondsis chinensis*). Jojoba "oil" is actually a liquid wax and doesn't become rancid.

Never use mineral oil!

The Quantity

Because they don't last for long periods of time, magical oils are made in small amounts. The following recipes use 1/8 cup of base oil.

The Blending

Place the base oil into a glass container, preferably one with a small opening at the top. Add the essential oils in the recommended amounts while visualizing the blend's intended purpose. After adding each ingredient, swirl the container clockwise until it has mixed with the oil. Do not stir.

Storage

Store magical oils as you would all essential oils—
away from heat, light and moisture, in dark-glassed,
labeled bottles.

Usage

Use according to intuition or as directed in each
recipe. Remember to visualize your needed goal while
using the oil.

One final word: these recipes create lightly-scented
oils. Don't expect the overpowering aromas that issue
from bottles of synthetic magical blends. Though these
fragrances don't knock you over (and burn your nos-
trils and brain), they are magically effective.

CASH FLOW OIL

1/8 cup Base oil
3 drops Vetivert
2 drops Patchouly
1 drop Ginger

Wear or anoint money before spending. Or, rub onto
green candles and burn while visualizing.

HEALING OIL

1/8 cup Base oil
7 drops Niaouli
4 drops Eucalyptus
2 drops Pine

Wear or anoint blue candles. Use in conjunction with
treatment!

LOVE OIL

1/8 cup Base oil
6 drops Ylang-Ylang
5 drops Palmarosa
3 drops Lavender
2 drops Geranium

Wear or add ten drops to the bath daily. Alternately, rub onto pink candles and burn while visualizing.

POWER OIL

1/8 cup Base oil
3 drops Patchouly
3 drops Black Pepper
1 drop Peppermint
1 drop Ginger
1 drop Orange

Wear to be in control of yourself and for extra physical or magical energy. An excellent oil for use in the morning when you wish to be ready to meet the day.

PROTECTION OIL

1/8 cup Base oil
5 drops Black Pepper
5 drops Petitgrain
2 drops Geranium

Anoint your body for protection while visualizing.

SPIRITUALITY OIL

1/8 cup Base Oil
7 drops Sandalwood
4 drops Cedarwood
1 drop Frankincense

Wear before all spiritual rituals.

TABLES OF SYNTHETIC AND GENUINE OILS

GENERALLY ARTIFICIAL OILS

The oils listed in the first table below are generally synthetic or natural bouquets, *i.e.*, blends composed of natural essential oils designed to approximate the scent of the oil after which it is named.

If you buy essential oils from the reliable companies listed in Appendix I you'll be fine. When purchasing from other outlets, keep this list in mind in determining whether an "essential oil" is genuine or not. Price as well as the other factors listed below should be taken in account.

ALMOND, SWEET (the genuine oil has no scent)
AMBERGRIS (synthetic)
APPLE BLOSSOM (synthetic)
BAYBERRY (easily imitated)
CARNATION (easily imitated; genuine essential oil unavailable)
CIVET (synthetic)
CLOVER (synthetic in use since 1898)
COCONUT (genuine oil has no "coconutty" scent)
FRANKINCENSE (often imitated)
GARDENIA (rarely available)
GINGER FLOWER (synthetic)
HELIOTROPE (easily imitated)
HONEY (an absolute of beeswax, which smells like honey, is produced but is unavailable in retail outlets)
HONEYSUCKLE (very costly)
HYACINTH (easily imitated)

JASMINE (very costly; if low priced, synthetic)
LILAC (unavailable)
LILY OF THE VALLEY (unavailable)
LOTUS (no true lotus oil exists)
MAGNOLIA (synthetic)
MELON (synthetic)
MIMOSA (unavailable)
MUSK (synthetic)
NARCISSUS (rarely available)
NEROLI (easily imitated; synthetic if not costly)
PLUMERIA (synthetic)
RASPBERRY (synthetic)
ROSE (if not costly, synthetic)
STEPHANOTIS (unavailable)
STRAWBERRY (synthetic)
TUBEROSE (rarely available)
VIOLET (costly)
WISTERIA (synthetic)

GENERALLY TRUE ESSENTIAL OILS

These oils are usually authentic. Once again, it can be difficult to determine this—some drug stores sell bottles of artificial cinnamon and clove oil, but at least they're marked as such. Let price, distributor and your nose be your judges! I have omitted those essential oils which should not be used by anyone except fully trained aromatherapists.

BERGAMOT
BLACK PEPPER
CAMOMILE

CARDAMOM
CEDARWOOD
CINNAMON
CLARY SAGE
CLOVE
CYPRESS
EUCALYPTUS
FENNEL
GRAPEFRUIT
JASMINE (only if costly)
LAVENDER
LEMON
LEMON BALM (but buy carefully; low-priced lemon balm essential oils, AKA Melissa, are often adulterated)
LEMON VERBENA
LIME
NEROLI (only if costly)
NIAOULI
NUTMEG
ORANGE
PATCHOULY
PEPPERMINT
PETITGRAIN
ROSE (if costly. Still may be adulterated)
ROSE GERANIUM
ROSEMARY
SANDALWOOD
SPEARMINT
TANGERINE
VETIVERT
YLANG-YLANG

I'm repeatedly warning you to buy only true essential oils for use in magical aromatherapy for these reasons:

    a. Synthetics don't work
    b. Synthetics can be hazardous to your health
    c. Synthetics aren't linked with the Earth

Playing guessing games when purchasing from unknown stores may result in garnering a collection of oils which are useless in magical aromatherapy.

If you value yourself and the Earth; if you wish to truly reap the benefits of magical aromatherapy, use only genuine, unadulterated essential oils.

HAZARDOUS ESSENTIAL OILS

The following essential oils have been determined to be hazardous and should be avoided or used with caution.

Many persons are susceptible to allergic reactions from essential oils which cause no problems for others. Pregnant women should especially avoid certain essential oils. Use all new essential oils with caution.

As an example, I recently received some Terebinth essential oil which is distilled from various pine resins. I inhaled it for several minutes and, soon afterward, experienced a severe allergic reaction. A check of the literature showed no history of terebinth's toxicity, so I chalked this up to an idiosyncratic (personal) allergic reaction.

No essential oils should be taken internally! Don't apply undiluted essential oils to the skin. Dilute with a carrier oil such as apricot kernel, hazelnut, almond, sesame, sunflower.

The information in this table has been collated from Robert Tisserand's *The Essential Oil Safety Data Manual*, from Appendix A of Patricia Davis' *Aromatherapy: An A-Z*, and from personal experience.

Remember: Essential oils are highly concentrated forms of the plants from which they're extracted. Most of the plant forms can be safely used, but it's difficult to predict allergic reactions.

Only those essential oils discussed in this book are listed here.

BASIL: Should not be used at all.

BERGAMOT: Phototoxic. If skin which has been anointed with bergamot essential oil is exposed to the Sun, severe sunburn may result.

CAMPHOR: Prolonged inhalation causes headache.

CINNAMON BARK AND LEAF: Skin irritants. Do not anoint or use in baths.

CLARY SAGE: Not to be used with alcohol. Prolonged inhalation may cause headache.

CLOVE BUD, STEM AND LEAF: Skin irritants. Do not anoint or use in baths.

FENNEL, BITTER: Irritant, causes epileptic attacks, not to be used by pregnant women.

FRANKINCENSE: May irritate skin.

HYSSOP: Causes epileptic attacks, possibly other problems. Do not use if pregnant.

LEMON: Irritant. Do not anoint or use in baths.

LEMON BALM: Irritant. Do not anoint or use in baths.

LEMON GRASS: Irritant. Do not anoint or use in baths.

LEMON VERBENA: Irritant. Do not anoint or use in baths.

MARJORAM: Not for use by pregnant women.

MUGWORT: Essential oil is hazardous and should not be used.

MYRRH: May cause skin irritation if anointed or used in baths. Do not use during pregnancy.

OREGANO: Irritant. Do not anoint or use in baths.

PENNYROYAL: Toxic. Do not use in any way! Pregnant women should especially avoid this essential oil.

PEPPERMINT: Skin irritant. Do not anoint or use in baths.

RUE: Dangerous. Do not use in any way!

SAGE (Dalmatian—*Salvia officinalis*): Toxic, epileptic attacks, not to be used by those with high blood pressure.

THYME: A hazardous, toxic essential oil. Skin irritant. Should not be used in essential oil form at all.

YLANG-YLANG: Prolonged inhalation may cause headache.

The most hazardous essential oils listed in this book are sage, mugwort, thyme, rue and pennyroyal. Most of the rest of them are safe for use (save for those special cases above).

When in doubt, use the fresh or dried plant form of the aroma in place of the essential oil.

APPENDIX I

ESSENTIAL OIL DISTRIBUTORS

AROMA VERA INC.
P. O. Box 3609
Culver City, CA 90231
(213) 280-0407

True essential oils, specially formulated aromatherapy blends and essential oil diffusors. Distributors of *The Handbook of Aromatherapy* by Marcel Lavabre. Send for free price list and brochure.

HERBAL ENDEAVOURS
3618 5. Emmons Ave.
Rochester Hills, MI 48063
(313) 852-0796

True essential oils and quality scented products. Books and diffusors are also available. Send $2.00 for catalog (refundable with first purchase).

LEYDET AROMATIC OILS
P. O. Box 2354
Fair Oaks, CA 95628
(916) 965-7546

True essential oils, diffusors, books, unique Zodiac blends and a complete line of aromatherapy products. Send $1.50 for price list and catalog.

LIFETREE AROMATIX
3949 Longridge Ave.
Sherman Oaks, CA 91423
(818) 986-0594 or (818) 789-2610

True essental oils from all over the world. Send $1.75 for catalog and price list.

ORIGINAL SWISS AROMATICS
P. O. Box 606
San Rafael, CA 94915
(415) 459-3998

True essential oils, blends and diffusors. Original Swiss Aromatics also offers a home study aromatherapy course—ask about it. Send $1.50 for price list.

WINDROSE AROMATICS
12629 N. Tatum Blvd. Ste. 611
Phoenix, AZ 85032

A complete line of essential oils and aromatic body care products, specializing in custom blends. Free catalogue and price list.

APPENDIX II

PLANT AND DRIED PLANT PRODUCT DISTRIBUTORS

Check local nurseries for live plants and bulbs, but don't be afraid to send away for those you can't find. The establishments listed below, which sell live plants, are completely reliable, as are those that vend dried herbs.

APHRODISIA
282 Bleeker St.
New York, NY 10018

A wide selection of dried herbs. Send $2.00 for catalog.

CAPRILAND'S HERB FARM
Silver Street
Coventry, CT 06238

Live aromatic plants, herb seeds and a delightful array of naturally scented herb products. Send SASE for their free catalog.

COMPANION PLANTS
724 7 N. Coolvill Ridge Rd.
Athens, OH 45701

Hundreds of rare and unusual plants and seeds (such as vanilla orchid and camphor tree). An astounding collection. Send $2.00 for catalog.

ENCHANTMENTS
341 E. 9th St.
New York, NY 1001)3

Dried herbs and herb books along with an enjoyable catalog of mystic items. Send $2.00 for catalog.

EYE OF THE CAT
3314 E. Broadway
Long Beach, CA 90803

One of the largest stocks of dried herbs anywhere. $5.00 gets you their herb catalog, which is virtually a book. If they don't have an herb, they might be able to get it for you.

PUNI PLANTS
Box 61487 Dept. SD
Honolulu, HI 96822

Tropical starter plants, including white ginger, plumeria, stephanotis and many others, shipped to every state in the country. With a minimum order, fresh flower leis are also available. Send $1.00 for full-color brochure and price list.

TAYLOR'S HERB GARDENS, INC.
1535 Lone Oak Road
Vista, CA 92084

Impressive collection of live plants including such rarities as the true bay tree. Their beautiful catalog, loaded with culinary recipes and full-color herb photographs, is available for $1.00.

APPENDIX III

AROMATHERAPY ORGANIZATIONS AND PUBLICATIONS

THE AMERICAN AROMATHERAPY
    ASSOCIATION
P. O. Box 1222
Fair Oaks, CA 95628

Publishes *Common Scents*, a quarterly periodical devoted to essential oils and aromatherapy, and holds annual conferences open to both members and non-members.

THE ASSOCIATION OF
    TISSERAND AROMATHERAPISTS
P. O. BOX 746
Hove
E. Sussex, BN3 3XA, ENGLAND

Conducts on-going research projects into essential oils.

THE INTERNATIONAL FEDERATION
   OF AROMATHERAPISTS
4 East Mearn Road
West Dulwich
London, SE2l 8HA, ENGLAND

Publishes a newsletter several times a year and acts as a clearing house for information regarding aromatherapy. Send a large self-addressed envelope along with several International Response Coupons for more information.

THE INTERNATONAL JOURNAL
   OF AROMATHERAPY
Aromatherapy Publications
10 Victoria Grove
Second Avenue
Hove
E. Sussex, BN3 2LJ, ENGLAND

"Promotes and exists for the benefit of all those with an interest in aromatherapy—with up-to-date information, news, research, case studies, and current happenings in Europe and the U.S.A. Current subscription information: UK and Europe: 15 pounds Sterling per year (four issues). Rest of the World: 18 pounds Sterling per year. Accepts Eurocheque, International Money Order or bank draft, drawn in Sterling on a London bank. They accept dollar checks from US subscribers as long as $5.00 is added to current sterling/dollar rate to cover bank handling charges. Make checks payable to "Aromatherapy Publications."

GLOSSARY

Italicized words defer to other related entries in this glossary.

ABSOLUTE: A perfumery product produced by solvent extraction. This is a complicated process entailing several stages, which eventuate in the production of the absolute. Jasmine absolute is one form. Compare with *Otto*.

ANAPHRODISIAC: A substance which lessens sexual arousal.

APHRODISIAC: A substance (such as an essential oil) which produces sexual arousal within its user.

AROMATHERAPY: The use of the healing properties of true *essential oils*. Conventional aromatherapy utilizes massage with diluted essential oils to correct imbalances in bodily energy and to directly treat existent conditions stemming from disordered physical, mental and emotional states. It is a non-magical practice.

B.C.E.: Before Common Era. The non-religious equivalent of B.C.

BIOELECTRICAL ENERGY: The natural energy which is created in our bodies by muscular contraction. It is available for use during *magic*. It is nurtured by personal power, which empowers our bodies and which we daily replenish with food, water, air, sunlight and other energy sources. Bioelectrical energy is the power used in all *magic*. In *magical aromatherapy*, we merge bioelectrical energy with the powers of fragrances and *essential oils*.

C.E.: Common Era. The non-religious equivalent of A.D.

CONSCIOUS MIND: The analytical, materially-based, rational half of the consciousness. The mind at work when we compute our taxes, theorize or struggle with ideas. Compare with *psychic mind*.

ELEMENTS, THE: Earth, Air, Fire, Water. These four energies are the building blocks of the universe. Everything that exists (or that has potential to exist) contains one or more of these non-physical energies. The elements are present within ourselves and are also at large in the world. They formed from the primal essence or power, Akasha.

ESSENTIAL OIL: Essential oils are fragrant, volatile substances produced by certain types of plants. In a sense, they are the "blood" of the plant, the manifestation of the life force which created it. In *magical aromatherapy*, the term usually refers to the liquids themselves, freed from the plants which created them. These natural aromas are the key tools of *aromatherapy*. They are also known as volatile oils and ethereals.

FOLK MAGIC: The practice of meshing *bioelectrical energy* with natural energies from plants, odors, stones, essential oils and other earthly products. The combined energies are moved to create a specific change.

MAGIC: The projection (movement) of subtle but natural energies to bring about needed change. This is a natural art which works with the forces of nature. It is not supernatural, "evil" or dangerous.

MAGICAL AROMATHERAPY: The utilization of aromatic plant materials, including essential oils, to produce specific changes. Natural fragrances are inhaled, the needed result is visualized and energy is moved through the agency of the *conscious mind*.

MEDITATION: Reflection, contemplation, turning inward toward the self or outward toward Deity or Nature. A quiet time in which the practitioner may dwell upon particular thoughts or symbols, or allow them to come unbidden.

OTTO: Rose otto (or attar) of rose is the essential oil which has been steam distilled from rose petals. It is much prized in cosmetic perfumery and in *aromatherapy*. Rose otto is purer than rose *absolute* and is more expensive. It is generally obtained from *Rosa damascena*.

PSYCHIC MIND: The subconscious or deep conscious mind, in which we receive psychic impulses. The psychic mind is at work when we sleep, dream, meditate and practice *magic*. It is our direct link with Nature and Deity. Intuition is a term used to describe psychic information which unexpectedly reaches the conscious mind.

RESINOID: A fragrant liquid created by solvent extraction of a resinous material such as a balsam or oleo-gum-resin. Benzoin is one example.

RITUAL: Ceremony. A specific form of movement, manipulation of objects or inner processes designed to produce the desired effects. In *magic*, ritual produces a specific state of consciousness which allows the practitioner to move energy toward needed goals. In *magical aromatherapy*, the simplest ritual involves *visualization* and inhalation of a specific natural aroma.

RITUAL CONSCIOUSNESS: The specific, alternate state of awareness necessary for the successful practice of *magic*. The practitioner achieves this through the use of *visualization* and *ritual*. It denotes a state in which the *conscious mind* and the *psychic mind* are attuned, in which the practitioner senses energies, gives them purpose and releases them toward the magical goal. It is a heightening of the senses, an awareness-expansion of the seemingly non-physical world, a linking with Nature.

SYNTHETIC "ESSENTIAL" OILS: Those fragrant oils which have not been obtained by steam distillation or cold expression from the naturally aromatic plant materials after which they are named. Synthetic scents are useless in both *magical aromatherapy* and its conventional cousin and shouldn't be used for these purposes under any circumstances. Compare with *Essential Oils*.

VISUALIZATION: The process of creating mental images. Magical visualization consists of forming images of needed goals during *ritual*. Visualization is also used to direct *bioelectrical energy* and the energies contained within natural fragrances during *magical aromatherapy* and other forms of *magic*. It is a function of the *conscious mind*.

BIBLIOGRAPHY

Aikman, Lonnelle, "Perfume, the Business of Illusion." *National Geographic*, April 1951, pp. 531-550.
A post-WWII look at the perfume industry, with excellent photographs of some of the plants from which essential oils are derived.

Arctander, Steffen, *Perfume and Flavor Materials of Natural Origin*. Elizabeth (New Jersey): Published by the author, 1960.
Scholarly discussions of the extraction of essential oils as well as articles detailing various scented plant materials. An invaluable (though non-magical) source of information regarding essential oils and aromatic plants.

Coles, William, *The Art of Simpling*. London, 1656. St. Catharine's (Ontario, Canada): Provoker Press, 1968.
Quaint tidbits of 300-year-old fragrance lore.

Culpeper, Nicholas, *The English Physician*. London: 1652. Reprint. Foulsham, ND.
Reprinted as *Culpepper's Herbal*, this work includes much old plant fragrance information.

Darby, William J. Paul Ghalioungui and Louis Grivetti, *Food: The Gift of Osiris*. Volume 2. London: Academic Press, 1977.

Fragments of Egyptian plant magic are included in this massive, authoritative 2-volume set.

Davis, Patricia, *Aromatherpy: An A-Z.* Saffron Walden (Essex, England): C. W. Daniel Company, 1988. This British import covers nearly every aspect of aromatherapy. Ms. Davis' expertise in this art shines through on each of the 398 pages. Some of her findings are controversial but the book is well worth reading.

Diamond, Denise, *Living With the Flowers: A Guide to Bringing Flowers into Your Daily Life.* New York: Quill, 1982. Chapter Six of this wonderful book discusses aromatherapy and flower essences. Beautiful artwork.

Dodoens, Rembert, *Kruydeboeck.* London: 1568. Much fascinating aromatic lore from another time and another place. Quoted at length in many other books.

Fox, Helen Morganthau, *Gardening With Herbs for Flavor and Fragrance.* New York: Macmillan, 1934. Much magical fragrance lore from ancient times.

Gattefosse, R. M. *Formulary of the Parisian Perfumer.* Villeurbanne-Lez-Lyon (France): Edition Parfumerie Moderne, 1923. An early work by the man who coined the term "aromatherapie." Originally published in 1907, this is the first edition in English. It describes types of essential oils, extraction processes and many other facets of pefumery. Because this book preceeded Mr. Gattefosse's pioneering work with aromatherapy, no information regarding the psychological and therapeutic effects of odors is included, but there is much else of interest.

Genders, Roy, *Growing Herbs as Aromatics.* New Canaan (Connecticut): Keats Publishing, 1977.
A short introduction to home cultivation of scented plants with some historical information.

Gerard, John, *The Herball, or Generall Historie of Plants.* London: 1597. Reprint. New York: Dover, 1975.
Hints of the powers of plant fragrances are scattered throughout this massive tome. Well worth reading for a genuine breath of 16th century life in England.

Gilmore, Melvin R., *Uses of Plants by the Indians of the Missouri River Region.* Thirty-Third Annual Report of the Bureau of American Ethnology. Washington: Government Printing Office, 1919.
American Indian plant perfume magic.

Grieve, M., *A Modern Herbal.* C. F. Leyel, editor. Two volumes. New York: Harcourt, Brace & Company, 1931. Reprint. New York: Dover, 1971.
A fascinating collection of botanical lore. The then-current knowledge of essential oils makes for stimulating reading. The author (and editor) included much lore concerning the ritual associations and uses of aromatic plant materials.

Heriteau, Jacqueline, *Potpourris and Other Fragrant Delights.* Harmondsworth (Middlesex, England): Penguin Books, 1986.
This small book contains curious lore regarding scented plants.

Hollingsworth, Buckner, *Flower Chronicles*. New Brunswick (New Jersey): Rutgers University Press, 1958.
Fascinating histories of flowers, including rose, saffron, nasturtium and many others. Entertaining reading.

Jacob, Dorothy, *A Witch's Guide to Gardening*. New York: Taplinger, 1965.
A delightful collection of plant lore.

Jellinek, Dr. Paul, *The Practice of Modern Perfumery*. Translated and revised by A. J. Krajkeman. New York: Interscience Publishers, 1954.
Part IV of this wonderful guide to cosmetic perfumery is titled "Perfumery, Cosmetics and Psychology." This 57-page section makes fascinating reading.

Junemann, Monika, *Enchanting Scents*. Wilmot (Wisconsin): Lotus Light, 1988.
Translated from the original German edition, this short book contains several unusual suggestions for using essential oils to change the inner self. Elemental and planetary information regarding essential oils is open to interpretation, and she does so in a most personal way.

Kamm, Minnie Watson, *Old-Time Herbs for Northern Gardens*. Boston: Little, Brown and Co., 1938.
A fine collection of ancient and contemporary herb lore, including the subtle effects of fragrant plants.

Kepler, Angela Kay, *Hawaiian Heritage Plants*. Honolulu: Oriental Publishing Co., 1983.
This wonderful book, packed with color photo-

graphs, contains some tidbits of Hawaiian perfume magic.

Krauss, Beatrice H., *Ethnobotany of the Hawaiians.* Harold L. Lyon Arboretum Lecture Number 5. Honolulu: Harold L. Lyon Arboretum, University of Hawaii, 1974.
This concise introduction to ancient Hawaiian plant use contains information on this peoples' creation of scented oils in pre-contact times.

Krutch, Joseph Wood, *Herbal.* Boston: David R. Godine, 1965.
This over-sized collection of old herbal lore contains much fragrance information.

Lautie, Raymond and Andre Passebecq, *Aromatherapy: The Use of Plant Essences in Healing.* Wellingborough (England): Thorsons Publishers Limited, 1979.
A short introduction to aromatherapy.

Lavabre, Marcel, "The Quality of Essential Oils—Clarifications and Definitions." *Common Scents* (the publication of the American Aromatherapy Association). Vol. 1. No. 1 (Fall, 1988).
Excellent, no-nonsense information relating to essential oils. Details some methods of determining true essential oils.

Lavabre, Marcel, *The Handbook of Aromatherapy.* Culver City (Calfornia): privately published, 1986.
An amazingly comprehensive introduction to conventional aromatherapy, containing information unavailable anywhere else. Mr. Lavabre details the emotional and spiritual effects of true essential oils

and, in an interesting chart, associates essential oils with the chakras and crystals (gemstones).

Leyel, C. F., *The Magic of Herbs*. New York: Harcourt, Brace and Company, 1926. Reprint. Toronto: Coles, 1981.
This classic work contains a wonderful chapter on perfumes and perfumers, including many recipes from ancient sources as well as information concerning classical Greek and Roman perfume use.

Loewe, Michael and Carmen Blacker, *Oracles and Divination*. Boulder (Colorado): Shambhala, 1981.
Ancient Babylonian uses of cedar during incense divination rituals.

Maple, Eric, *The Magic of Perfume*. Weiser: New York, 1973.
This short booklet includes historical as well as contemporary information concerning the effects of scent on human beings.

McDonald, Marie A., *Ka Lei: The Leis of Hawaii*. Honolulu and Waipahu (Hawaii): Topgallant Publishing Co. and Press Pacifica, 1978.
A glorious, full-color guide to this fascinating subject, *Ka Lei* includes ancient ritual uses of fragrant flowers

Meyer, Clarence, *Fifty Years of the Herbalist Almanac*. Glenwood (Illinois): Meyerbooks, 1977.
A treasury of ancient and modern herbal lore, including that of American Indians—" the race that lived with nature." Invaluable for all aspects of herbalism. Scent magic abounds.

Moldenke, Harold, *Plants of the Bible*. Waltham (Massachusetts): Chronica Botanica Company, 1952.
Background information on aromatic plants in the ancient world.

Morgan, Harry T., *Chinese Symbols and Superstitions*. South Pasadena (California): P. D. and Ione Perkins, 1942.
Chinese symbolism of flowering plants is included in this fascinating work.

Morris, Edwin T., *Fragrance: The Story of Perfume from Cleopatra to Chanel*. New York: Charles Scribner's Sons, 1984.
A comprehensive, authoritative history of the uses of scented plant materials from the earliest times to the present day. Heavily illustrated. Footnotes and an extensive bibliography.

Murphey, Edith Van Allen, *Indian Uses of Native Plants*. Fort Bragg (California): Mendocino County Historical Society, 1959.
A stimulating collection of Indian ethnobotany, including plant magic, garnered from living informants in the 1940s.

Poucher, William A., *Perfumes, Cosmetics and Soaps*. Three Volumes. Princeton: D. Van Nostrand and Co., Inc., 1958.
Discussions of the main aromatic plants and essential oils. It lacks magical information.

Rose, Jeanne, *Herbs and Things: Jeanne Rose's Herbal*. New York: Grosset & Dunlap, 1974.
Ms. Rose includes magical and medicinal aromatic information in this classic work.

Rose, Jeanne, *Jeanne Rose's Modern Herbal.* New York: Perigee, 1987.
Chapter 12, "Aromatherapy and Color," makes for fascinating reading.

Thompson, C. J. S., *The Mystery and Lure of Perfume.* Philadelphia: J. B. Lippincott, 1927.
This work is solely dedicated to ritual and magical uses of natural aromatics. Several chapters discuss incense and perfume use from antiquity up to the 1920s.

Tisserand, Maggie, *Aromatherapy For Women.* Wellingborough (Northamptonshire, England): Thorson's, 1985.
A charming guide to utilizing essential oils for everyday problems, with some surprising suggestions.

Tisserand, Robert, *Aromatherapy for Everyone.* Harmondsworth (Middlesex, England): Penguin Books, 1988. Released in the U.S. as *Aromatherapy to Tend and Heal the Body.* Wilmot (Wisconsin): Lotus Light, 1989.
Mr. Tisserand's newest book is a welcome addition to the literature. It is a comprehensive, easily-read introduction to conventional (holistic) aromatherapy, stressing its history, current applications and effectiveness. This wonderful book should be used with the below title.

Tisserand, Robert, *The Art of Aromatherapy.* New York: Destiny Books, 1977.
An invaluable guide to aromatherapy by an acknowledged master. Detailed, informative, written

in Mr. Tisserand's lively style, it is must reading.

Tisserand, Robert, *Essential Oil Safety Data Manual*. Brighton (Sussex, England): The Association of Tisserand Aromatherapists, 1985.
This privately published, limited-edition book is the accepted resource outlining the dangers of certain essential oils. I extensively utilized this information while writing this book. Well-researched, documented and highly recommended. Portions of this work were included in Mr. Tisserand's *Aromatherapy for Everyone*. A new edition has recently been published.

Trueman, John, *The Romantic Story of Scent*. Garden City (New York): Doubleday and Company, 1975.
A richly illustrated history of aromatic materials, this book was unique in including "scratch and sniff" samples of 18 natural (and, sadly, synthetic) scents (such as lavender, clove and patchouly) on the dust jacket. Today, 14 years later, they still release their respective scents.

Valnet, Jean, *The Practice of Aromatherapy*. Rochester (Vermont) Destiny Books, ND.
A classic guide to the physiological and psychological effects of essential oils. Written by a famed M.D., this is heavy reading. However, a medical glossary explains most of the specialized terms.

Verrill, A. Hyatt, *Perfumes and Spices*. New York: L. C. Page and Co., 1940.
A detailed account of perfumery, with many interesting tips on blending oils and recipes (non-

magical in nature, of course).

Wall, O. A., *Sex and Sex Worship*. St. Louis: C. V. Mosby Company, 1919.
This fascinating, monumental account includes a section titled "Gratification of the Senses." In it, Dr. Wall discusses the use of incense among ancient peoples, perfume in general and the sense of smell as it was understood in 1919. In a curious section, he makes a detailed investigation of the natural odors of hygenic, healthy women. Some of this information seems to have been utilized by Jellinek (see above).

Wheelright, Edith, *Medicinal Plants and their History*. New York: Dover, 1974.
Mesopotamian fragrance magic.

Wilder, Louise Beebe, *The Fragrant Garden*. New York: Dover, 1972.
Originally published in 1932 under the title *The Fragrant Path*, this is a consuming, loving rendition of a scented garden between the covers of a book. Excerpts from ancient works discuss the "vertues" of scented plants. Much lore.

INDEX

STAY IN TOUCH

On the following pages you will find books on related subjects. Your book dealer stocks most of these and will stock new Llewellyn titles as they become available.

You may also request our bimonthly catalog, *Llewellyn's New Worlds of Mind and Spirit.* A sample copy is free, and it will continue coming to you at no cost as long as you are an active mail customer. Or you may subscribe for just $7.00 in the U.S.A. and Canada ($20.00 overseas, first class mail). Many bookstores also have *New Worlds* available to their customers. Ask for it.

Llewellyn's New Worlds of Mind and Spirit
P.O. Box 64383-129, St. Paul, MN 55164-0383, U.S.A.
* * *

TO ORDER BOOKS AND TAPES

You may order books directly from the publisher by sending full price in U.S. funds, plus $3.00 for postage and handling for orders *under* $10.00; $4.00 for orders *over* $10.00. There are no postage and handling charges for orders over $50.00. Postage and handling rates are subject to change. We ship UPS whenever possible. Delivery guaranteed. Provide your street address as UPS does not deliver to P.O. Boxes. Allow 4-6 weeks for delivery. UPS to Canada requires a $50.00 minimum order. Orders outside the U.S.A. and Canada: Airmail—add retail price of book; add $5.00 for each non-book item (tapes, etc.); add $1.00 per item for surface mail. For customer service, call 1-612-291-1970.

FOR GROUP STUDY AND PURCHASE

Our special quantity price for a minimum order of five copies of *Magical Aromatherapy* is $11.85 cash-with-order. This price includes postage and handling within the United States. Minnesota residents must add 6.5% sales tax. For additional quantities, please order in multiples of five. For Canadian and foreign orders, add postage and handling charges as above. Mail orders to:

LLEWELLYN PUBLICATIONS
P.O. Box 64383-129, St. Paul, MN 55164-0383, U.S.A.

Prices subject to change without notice.

EARTH POWER
by Scott Cunningham

This is a book of folk magic—the magic of the common people. As such, it is different from nearly every other published work on the subject. This book is for the people of the Earth. The practices are so easy as placing a leaf in a north wind. The ritual is married to the forces of Nature. This is natural magic rediscovered.

This book can not only help you learn these natural magical methods, but it can also put you in touch with the planet that nurtures you, and gives you spells for every purpose including: weather magic, dieting, love spells, divination, meditation, protection and much more. *Earth Power* is folk magic—the magic of common people that does not need years of study, expensive paraphernalia and long rituals filled with meaningless words. Instead, it uses the *innate* magical powers of nature. Scott has uncovered magical secrets from centuries ago so that you can use them—to help yourself and loved ones—today.

0-87542-121-0, 153 pages, 5¼ x 8, illus., softcover.　**$8.95**

MAGICAL HERBALISM—The Secret Craft of the Wise
by Scott Cunningham

In *Magical Herbalism*, certain plants are prized for the special range of energies or powers they possess. This book unites the powers of plants and man to produce, and direct, change in accord with human will and desire.

This is the Magic of amulets and charms, sachets and herbal pillows, incenses and scented oils, simples and infusions and anointments. It is a magic to enjoy as we look to the Earth to rediscover our roots and make inner connections with the world of Nature.

This is the Magic of Enchantment . . . of word and gesture to shape the images of mind and channel the energies of the herbs. It is a Magic for *everyone*—for the herbs are easily and readily obtained, the tools are familiar or easily made, and the technology that of home and garden.

This book includes step-by-step guidance to the preparation of herbs and to their compounding in incense and oils, sachets and amulets, simples and infusions, with simple rituals and spells for every purpose.

0-87542-120-2, 243 pages, 5¼ x 8, illus., softcover　**$7.95**